Borderline Personality Disorder

An evidence-based guide for generalist mental health professionals

Anthony W. Bateman
Consultant Psychiatrist and Psychotherapist, Barnet,
Enfield, and Haringey Mental Health NHS Trust
Visiting Professor, University College, London
Consultant, Anna Freud Centre, London, UK

and

Roy Krawitz
Consultant Psychiatrist and DBT Therapist,
Waikato District Health Board
Honorary Clinical Senior Lecturer, Auckland University,
New Zealand

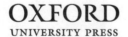

OXFORD
UNIVERSITY PRESS

OXFORD
UNIVERSITY PRESS

Great Clarendon Street, Oxford, OX2 6DP,
United Kingdom

Oxford University Press is a department of the University of Oxford.
It furthers the University's objective of excellence in research, scholarship,
and education by publishing worldwide. Oxford is a registered trade mark of
Oxford University Press in the UK and in certain other countries

First Edition published in 2013

Impression: 1

British Library Cataloguing in Publication Data

Data available

ISBN 978–0–19–964420–9

Printed and bound in Great Britain by
Clays Ltd, St Ives plc

Preface

Over the past two decades considerable progress has been made in developing specialist psychosocial treatments for borderline personality disorder (BPD) and yet the majority of people with BPD receive treatment within generalist mental health services rather than specialist treatment centres. It turns out that this is no bad thing. Many of the lessons learned from the development of specialist treatments for BPD now inform general psychiatric care and we can confidently say that treatment of people with BPD by generalist clinicians is no longer necessarily suboptimal and may in fact, in some contexts, be equal to specialist treatments as long as certain principles are followed and interventions are skillfully implemented. This is why this book came about.

There is increasing evidence that well-organized and skillful generalist psychiatric treatments for BPD, at least when used as comparators to specialist interventions in research trials, are strikingly effective. We discuss the evidence for this statement in Chapter 2. One of four published and manualized generalist psychiatric treatments used in research—structured clinical management (SCM)—forms the core of this book. SCM was used as a control treatment in a randomized controlled trial investigating the effectiveness of mentalization-based treatment. Patients who received SCM fared well on all measures. SCM follows organizational and clinical principles considered by experts to be important in the treatment of people with BPD. Rather than requiring complex specialist techniques, SCM employs interventions already in use by generalist mental health clinicians. The book is a development of the SCM manual used in the randomized controlled trial and we have extended the information for clinicians, added further suggestions of interventions, and reviewed some of the other literature on generalist psychiatric treatments.

This is not a book by specialists telling generalists what to do. We firmly believe that generalists are highly skilled clinicians and are able to deliver treatment that is not necessarily within the capability of the specialist. We wrestled with the terms "general" versus "generalist" clinicians for the book, eventually choosing generalist despite it being a rather ungainly word in the hope that we would avoid being considered patronizing or insulting. Generalist emphasizes the breadth of the clinician's skill and implies, accurately in our view, an ability to implement a range of techniques according to specific principles and to integrate them into a coherent treatment endeavour. This book speaks to those skills. It outlines the principles to be followed when treating people with BPD in mental health services and details a range of effective techniques that can be used by generalist clinicians in everyday practice without extensive additional training.

Although the book is organized around the research manual for SCM, it is more than that. It is a comprehensive, best-practice clinical guideline for the treatment of BPD in generalist mental health services. The structure of the book is straightforward. First, we provide considerable information about BPD; second, we discuss the evidence base for and the characteristics of the manualized generalist psychiatric treatments that have been tested in research trials. This is followed by chapters about the general and specific clinical components of SCM, with an emphasis on practical implementation. Finally, we outline our approach to involving families and summarize our top ten tips for effective interventions in the hope that clinicians will go beyond SCM, both safely and effectively, as they grow increasingly confident about treating people with BPD.

We first encountered people with BPD when working as trainees in generalist mental health services and were immediately aware of our lack of understanding of their problems and the limited knowledge we had to draw on to help them. Despite these experiences, or perhaps because of them, we both embarked on a career working with people with BPD, gradually sharing our experience and knowledge, mostly gleaned from our clients/patients, with other mental health clinicians.

That observation raises the issues of who *we*, the authors, are, coming as we do from opposite sides of the globe. We both have considerable psychiatric experience working in public health services. One of us (AB) is a psychiatrist with dynamic leanings whilst the other (RK) is a psychiatrist with behavioral orientation. We hope that as a team we have enough in common to provide a unified view, enough difference to add breadth and plurality to our exposition, and adequate open-mindedness not to be too reverential to our favored approaches. On the whole our collaboration has run smoothly and it has become apparent that our differences are narrower than might be assumed from our distinctive perspectives. Certainly we think that combining our knowledge and experience has strengthened the book.

We hope that the book is reader- and clinician-friendly; parts are set out so that they can be easily copied to support treatment and we give a liberal sprinkling of consumer comments to illustrate many of our points. We are only too aware of the many faults of omission in the book. We have not tackled in detail the issues of ethnicity, class, social context, and gender in relation to BPD. Apropos of the latter, like many contemporary authors we have been stymied by the problem of pronouns, but, in the end, decided to mix and match, sometimes using the possibly less grammatically obtrusive, but patriarchal, "he" and at other times "she." For the most part we have avoided the grammatically clumsy "they" with a singular verb and the clumsy "s/he". We had a similar struggle with a decision on whether to use the terms "client," "service user," "consumer" or "patient". "Client" is considered to imply equality and collaboration whilst "patient" is often taken to indicate a hierarchical interaction. So, believing that neither portrayal is necessarily accurate, we have used both "client" and "patient." We have also used "consumer" when we report comments given to us by people with BPD, or their families, where they had experience of the services and treatments. We have avoided "service user," which lacked finesse.

It is our hope that this book will be a modest contribution to improving generalist psychiatric treatments for people with BPD. Above all we hope that the information and clinical suggestions contained in the book will help generalist clinicians approach people with BPD not only with increasing confidence about being able to offer effective treatment, but also with a level of commitment and seriousness that many clients have arguably been deprived of in the past both in their personal lives and in their contact with services.

Anthony W. Bateman
Roy Krawitz
London, UK, and Auckland/Waikato,
New Zealand, July 2012

Contents

1 Borderline personality disorder *1*

2 Generalist psychiatric treatments for borderline personality disorder: the evidence base and common factors *34*

3 Structured clinical management: general treatment strategies *56*

4 Structured clinical management: core treatment strategies *80*

5 Structured clinical management: team strategies *112*

6 Structured clinical management: inpatient treatment and prescribing *124*

7 Family and friends *143*

8 Top ten additional resource-efficient treatment strategies *174*

Epilogue *203*

References *205*

Index *223*

Chapter 1

Borderline personality disorder

Summary

- Community lifetime prevalence of BPD is 1% (Grant et al., 2008; Schwartz, 1991), with equal rates of males and females in the Grant et al. study (2008).
- 70% of those diagnosed are female (Schwartz, 1991).
- It is likely that males are underrepresented and underdiagnosed in mental health settings and more likely to be found (but not diagnosed) in substance-use centers and in the justice system.
- 40–70% of those diagnosed have a history of past sexual abuse.
- 46% of people with BPD have a history of being victims of adult violence (Zanarini et al., 1999).
- Prevalence of people with BPD is estimated at community clinics to be about 11% and 20% in inpatient units (Swartz, Blazer, George, & Winfield, 1990).
- 75% of people with BPD have a history of having self-harmed on at least one occasion (Dubo, Zanarini, Lewis, & Williams, 1997).
- Most experts in the field accept BPD as a valid recognizable condition.
- For a DSM-IV-TR diagnosis of BPD, five or more of the criteria listed in DSM-IV-TR are required.
- It is important that diagnosis is only one part of understanding the unique individuality of the person.
- It is important that the diagnosis is integrated with other ways of understanding the person.
- Severe dissociation and persistent self-harm are often discriminating features in making a diagnosis.
- Co-occurring Axis 1 and II conditions are the norm.
- Suicide rates in older studies were 10% and are lower now with better treatments.

- There is considerable overlap between BPD and depression, dysthymia, bipolar affective disorder, and psychotic phenomena.
- Biological and psychological factors may be causal, with each client having a unique pathway to developing the disorder.
- The function of self-harm is almost always to decrease distress, and can be categorized by decreasing distress directly or by decreasing distress indirectly by effects on people in the environment.
- Naturalistic studies show that people with BPD improve over time, with high rates of remission lasting longer than 4 years (86%) and with low rates of relapse (33% over 8 years) at 10-year follow-up.
- Psychotherapy is the recommended treatment, with medication as an adjunct.
- There are now nearly 20 randomized controlled trials demonstrating the effectiveness of psychological treatments.
- There is a modest research base providing evidence of the effectiveness of high-quality generalist treatments.

History

The term "borderline personality disorder" (BPD) was initially suggested in the 1930s by clinicians to identify a group of clients who did not fit into the usual categorizations of "neurotic," including what we now refer to as anxiety and depressive disorders, or "psychotic," including what we now refer to as bipolar disorder and schizophrenia. Clinicians found that there was a group of clients who, descriptively, in most ways fitted the "neurotic" category except that they did not respond to the usual treatments at the time. The term "borderline" referred to the belief at the time that this group of people were on the "border" between "neurotic" and "psychotic." Whilst some people with BPD do have occasional psychotic or psychotic-like experiences, this definition of BPD, being on the "border," no longer applies, but the term has become ingrained. This might change as a result of controversial modifications to the classification of personality disorders being proposed by both the work group for the new *Diagnostic and Statistical Manual 5* (Skodol et al., 2011) and the personality disorder development group of the *International Classification of Diseases* 11th revision (Tyrer et al., 2011). In both classifications BPD will not be a discreet category of personality disorder, much to the disquiet of many experts (Bateman, 2011; Gunderson, 2010).

There was discussion in the 1970s of BPD as a variant of schizophrenia, in the 1980s as a variant of depression, in the 1990s as a variant of post-traumatic disorder, and since then as a variant of bipolar affective disorder. We have always seen and continue to see BPD rather as a dimensional disorder and variant of normal personality. This latter view is likely to be reflected in the DSM-V diagnostic system.

For the majority of the 20th century, treatment outcomes for people diagnosed with BPD were generally poor. Clinicians and research scientists turned their energies and interests in other directions. In the late 20th century, clinicians began successfully modifying and adapting their treatments, resulting in improved outcomes for people diagnosed with BPD. Professional and scientific interest in the condition soared and continues to grow.

The first scientific evidence of effective treatment was published in 1991, representing a major turning point in the treatment of people with BPD. Since 1991, there have been numerous further reports of effective treatment, with publications growing at an increased rate. People with BPD are now recognized as having a disabling condition that is often extremely severe and warranting compassionate and effective treatment.

Epidemiology

The most recent and very large (35,000 people) epidemiological study in the USA showed a lifetime prevalence rate of 5.9% (Grant et al., 2008). Earlier studies showed a prevalence of 1–1.8% (Swartz, Balzer, George, & Winfield, 1990; Widiger & Weissman, 1991).

As yet an unanswered question is whether the number of people meeting criteria for BPD would be less in cultures where strong family and extended family connections remain. The movement of people to cities, increased family mobility, loss of the small village culture, and lessened family and extended family connections are all sociocultural factors that might plausibly increase the likelihood of people developing BPD. Nuclear families might not have the same protection as the small village and extended family culture. Anecdotal evidence suggests the prevalence in westernized countries may also be directly correlated with the ratio of the earnings gap between the poorest and richest people, with Norway having the lowest prevalence and the USA the greatest prevalence.

Seventy-five percent of those diagnosed are female (Swartz, Blazer, et al., 1990); but there was no difference in rates in Grant et al.'s 2008 community epidemiological study. It is likely that males are underrepresented and underdiagnosed in mental health settings and more likely to be found (but not diagnosed) in substance-use centers and in the justice system. Black et al. (2007) found 29.5% of recently imprisoned people met the criteria for BPD. Forty to seventy percent of those diagnosed have a history of past sexual abuse (Herman, Perry, & van der Kolk, 1989; Ogata, Silk, & Goodrich, 1990; Widiger & Frances, 1989). Zanarini et al. (1999) report 46% of people with BPD in their study as having a history of being victims of adult violence (physical and/or sexual assault). People meeting the criteria are well represented in mental health facilities, with estimates of 11% at community clinics and 20% in inpatient units (Swartz, Balzer, et al., 1990). Seventy-five percent of people with BPD have a history of having self-harmed on at least one occasion (Dubo et al., 1997).

Diagnosis

Most experts in the field accept BPD as a valid recognizable condition and this is acknowledged in BPD being a DSM-IV-TR diagnosis. For a DSM-IV-TR diagnosis of BPD, one needs to have five or more of the criteria listed in DSM-IV-TR and the criteria need to be pervasive (wide range of personal/ social situations) and enduring (long-standing, with onset usually in adolescence or early adulthood and stable over time), and lead to significant distress or impairment in functioning. If a person meets three or four of the nine BPD criteria, and if these features are enduring and causing significant life problems, they could be said to have BPD traits.

A positive diagnosis of BPD is ideally made without it being a diagnosis of exclusion (when all other diagnoses have been tried and eliminated, or there is a failure to respond to medications). Avoiding making a diagnosis to avoid clinician and client negativity is now inappropriate given the positive, natural course of the disorder and the availability of effective treatment. On the other hand, the diagnosis of BPD may only become apparent after a longitudinal pattern, not readily recognizable at initial cross-sectional presentation, becomes more clearly illuminated during treatment.

People with substance-use conditions often have unstable lives due to the direct physiological destabilizing effects of the substance and sometimes due to associated behaviors such as engaging in criminal activity to fund the purchase of substances. As such, we need to be a little cautious making a BPD diagnosis in the presence of a substance-use disorder. However, about 50% of people with a BPD diagnoses have a lifetime history of alcohol or other drug problems (Swartz, Balzer, et al., 1990). Making both diagnoses can be very helpful.

BPD is a diagnosis most often applied only to adults. As adolescence is a period when many BPD features occur as part of normal adolescent development, many clinicians tend to prefer not to make the diagnosis in teenage years. The terms "emerging" and "subsyndromal" BPD are sometimes used to describe young people who are having problems related to BPD features but who are too young to be sure that they will have the condition as they enter adulthood. Many experts working with adolescents are confident of being able to diagnose BPD where the behaviors are florid, and they emphasize the value of making an early diagnosis so as to be able to initiate effective treatments before the person and mental health system get locked into mutually reinforcing ineffective behaviors. Chanen et al.'s (2008) randomized controlled trial demonstrated that it is possible to identify and effectively treat adolescents with full or subsyndromal BPD, thereby also going some way to alleviate fears of iatrogenic dangers of diagnosis in adolescence (Chanen, Jovev, & Jackson, 2007).

To diagnose or not to diagnose?

More important than diagnosis, we encourage understanding of the condition called BPD so that we can put in place effective treatments for the condition. The disadvantages of any mental health diagnosis can potentially include a failure to recognize the uniqueness and humanity of the person with the condition. Disadvantages specific to BPD potentially could be clinician and client negativity where the diagnosis triggers pessimism. Neither of these needs to occur. Diagnosis can serve as a guide to effective compassionate treatment, with clinicians and clients sourcing information about the condition, developing a common language, and researching into the condition and into effective treatments. Increasingly people with BPD are being told about the diagnosis, enabling clinician and client to join together as a true collaborative team, each with their individual responsibilities.

Consumer comment

As a registered nurse trained in the early 1980s I had absorbed the profession's negative perception of people with BPD at the time, which meant that when I was finally diagnosed with BPD that I was mortified to be seen to be one of those "terrible" people. Being given a correct diagnosis, however, resulted for the first time in my receiving appropriate support and treatment. Being given an accurate diagnosis was the major turning point in my life, eventually allowing me to leave BPD behind and live the fulfilling life I do now. (Jackson, personal communication)

Alternative names used to describe BPD

There have been explorations of alternative names for BPD. "Complex post-traumatic stress disorder" (Herman, 1992) acknowledges in the name the role of past trauma, but is not inclusive of those for whom trauma is not a feature. "Emotion regulation disorder" and "emotional intensity disorder" highlight the central feature of heightened emotional sensitivity and reactivity. We like the term "emotion regulation disorder," if not as a diagnostic name, then as a way of understanding the condition and as a way of thinking to aid treatment and recovery, although it fails to highlight the interpersonal sensitivity that many feel is at the core of the disorder. Perhaps "emotional and interpersonal regulation disorder" might be better, albeit rather a mouthful! To some extent the new classification systems are trying to focus more on these core areas of personality disorder.

The International Classification of Diseases (ICD) proposal is to classify personality disorders according to whether one is present or absent. Personality disorder is based on an assessment of a person's capacity to function interpersonally. If present, one of five levels of severity is given to the individual. Only then does the clinician determine the main aspects of the personality disturbance using five major domains, namely asocial, dissocial, anxious dependent, emotionally unstable, and obsessional/anankastic. People with BPD are likely, therefore, to be classified as personality disorder, severe, with anxious/dependent and emotionally unstable characteristics.

The new DSM proposal is more complex. Personality disorder is defined according to an assessment of interpersonal function and self along with the presence of pathological personality traits. Once the level of interpersonal function has been defined, the clinician decides if one of six defined types is present. Currently these are antisocial, avoidant, borderline, narcissistic, obsessive-compulsive, and schizotypal so the term "borderline" will remain but become a subcategory in a dimensional classification system.

Diagnostic criteria

The current criteria in the DSM-IV-TR for BPD are well known. Patients with BPD show a pervasive pattern of instability of interpersonal relationships, self-image and affects, and marked impulsivity beginning by early adulthood and present in a variety of contexts. Five out of nine criteria have to be present for a formal diagnosis. The nine criteria are:

1. frantic efforts to avoid real or imagined abandonment
2. pattern of unstable and intense interpersonal relationships
3. identity disturbance

4. impulsivity

5. recurrent suicidal behavior, gestures or threats, or self mutilating behavior

6. affective instability

7. chronic feelings of emptiness

8. inappropriate intense anger or difficulty controlling anger

9. transient, stress-related paranoid ideation or severe dissociative symptoms.

DSM-IV-TR diagnostic criteria for borderline personality disorder

The DSM-IV-TR diagnostic criteria for borderline personality disorder are detailed in the *Diagnostic and Statistical Manual of Mental Disorders* (American Psychiatric Association, 2000) and are reprinted here with permission.

> A pervasive pattern of instability of interpersonal relationships, self-image and affects, and marked impulsivity beginning by early adulthood and present in a variety of contexts, as indicated by five (or more) of the following:
>
> (1) frantic efforts to avoid real or imagined abandonment. Note: Do not include suicidal or self-mutilating behavior covered in Criterion 5
>
> (2) a pattern of unstable and intense interpersonal relationships characterized by alternating between extremes of idealization and devaluation
>
> (3) identity disturbance: markedly and persistently unstable self-image or sense of self
>
> (4) impulsivity in at least two areas that are potentially self damaging (e.g., spending, sex, substance abuse, reckless driving, binge eating). Note: Do not include suicidal or self-mutilating behavior covered in Criterion 5
>
> (5) recurrent suicidal behavior, gestures or threats or self mutilating behavior
>
> (6) affective instability due to a marked reactivity of mood (e.g., intense episodic dysphoria, irritability or anxiety usually lasting a few hours and only rarely more than a few days)
>
> (7) chronic feelings of emptiness
>
> (8) inappropriate intense anger or difficulty controlling anger (e.g., frequent displays of temper, constant anger, recurrent physical fights)
>
> (9) transient, stress-related paranoid ideation or severe dissociative symptoms.

We have adapted the formal diagnostic criteria into a series of initial common-language screening questions we ask our clients:

1. Are you scared of rejection and abandonment, and being left all alone?

2. Are your relationships with your friends and family unstable?

3. Do you see things as either all good or all bad, 100% right or 100% wrong, or in absolute terms, e.g. everybody is…; all men are…?

4. Do you have trouble knowing who you are and what is important to you?

5. Do you impulsively do things which might damage yourself in some way?

6. Do you self-harm (intentional harm to body, including overdoses) or behave in a suicidal manner?

7. Do you have mood swings that could change quickly?

8. Do you feel empty and feel you need others to fill you up and make you whole?

9. Do you get excessively angry in a manner that is to your own detriment?

10. Do you numb out (dissociate) or sometimes feel overly suspicious or paranoid when stressed?

Elaboration of DSM-IV-TR criteria with view to understanding

Criterion 1: Frantic efforts to avoid real or imagined abandonment

Does your client cling to others or become desperate when someone seems to reject them? If for whatever reason (biological predisposition, psychological trauma) our clients as children did not have regular experiences of being securely attached to important people who would be able to assist them deal with their intense distress, it is likely that they will bring this experience into their adult world, believing that important people may not be there for them when they need them. They might fear being left alone and helpless to face what they believe is a tough harsh world. This fear of abandonment will understandably result in "frantic efforts to avoid real or imagined abandonment."

"Frantic efforts to avoid real or imagined abandonment" may take forms from being as helpless as possible to expressing drastic thoughts of what will happen if left feeling abandoned. These behaviors might encourage some people to engage, which may prevent abandonment, especially in the short term. However, these behaviors may actually drive people away or be destructive to the very relationship that the individual is trying to protect. Sometimes the person with BPD may themselves end the relationship as a way of getting in first, thereby avoiding the imagined inevitable abandonment.

Consumer comment

I often caused myself a lot of distress by ending friendships or relationships if someone seemed angry or unhappy with me because I believed they were going to walk out of my life, even if they were only a little angry with me. It was really important to me that I took control and walked away first. I lost a lot of relationships like this (Krawitz & Jackson, 2008).

Criterion 2: A pattern of unstable and intense interpersonal relationships characterized by alternating between extremes of idealization and devaluation

Does your client put others on an elevated platform, seeing them as perfect—or possibly perfect—saviors and everything that they had wished for and later find themselves full of contempt for the person and hating them? Young children often relate to important people in an all-or-nothing manner, seeing them one moment as perfect before, after a real or imagined slight, raging against them and hating them. Without the right circumstances, children might not develop and mature into adults that see people as having both desirable and less desirable attributes. This idealizing and devaluation will be very hard on your client and the people with whom they are in relationships. Identity disturbance (Criterion 3), impulsivity (Criterion 4), affective instability (Criterion 6), and difficulty controlling anger (Criterion 8) will contribute to unstable and perhaps turbulent relationships.

Consumer comment

I was an expert at putting people on a pedestal. I would meet somebody and they were the answer to my dreams. Then they would turn out to be only human after all and my image of the person was dashed—they were the most dreadful person in the world and how could I have been such a bad judge of character? (Krawitz, 2008).

Criterion 3: Identity disturbance: markedly and persistently unstable self-image or sense of self

Does your client ask questions of themselves like, "Who am I, what do I want from life, and what do I want to do with my life?" Does your client search continuously for answers to these questions only to find that when they think they are getting to know what they want from life that they lose interest? This may be an outcome of unharnessed emotional intensity or it might be an understandable searching for what makes sense to them in a world that has, to date, not made that much sense. If their previous experience of emotions has been very painful, they might have coped by shutting out/avoiding as much of their feelings and emotions as they could. This may have worked for our clients to some degree in decreasing distress in the short term. Deprived of the important information that emotions give people, this may have had the effect of leaving people with BPD feeling empty and uncertain about what they want from life.

Consumer comment

For most of my life I had no idea who I was. I would suck up the identities of those around me. I would meet someone and as mentioned above would think they were the perfect example of the human species. I would hang out with them, and do the things they did. At various points I was an active left-of-centre political party member, right-of-centre political party member, had short hair, long hair, liked country music, then rock, loved being a nurse, hated being a nurse, and on it went (Krawitz & Jackson, 2008).

Criterion 4: Impulsivity in at least two areas that are potentially self-damaging (e.g., spending, sex, substance abuse, reckless driving, binge eating). Note: do not include suicidal or self-mutilating behavior covered in Criterion 5

Impulsive behaviors may arise for our clients when they are so distressed that they will do virtually anything to feel even a little bit better even if this only lasts a short while and even if it has serious long-term consequences. It is much like, and includes, being addicted to substances like alcohol or heroin that briefly help people feel better in the short term but have serious negative consequences. If our lives are full of pain and we have yet to learn effective ways of dealing with our distress, then impulsive behaviors are understandable, and very likely. Impulsive behaviors may include gambling, binge eating, driving recklessly, sex that is regretted, excessive spending, assault, alcohol use, and other substance use.

Consumer comment

For many years, spending was something that gave me instant gratification. If I was feeling distressed, I would go shopping—frequently buying things I never used and often not being able to pay essential bills. I would have some sense in the back of my mind that I might regret this later, but the need to instantly feel better was all-encompassing (Krawitz & Jackson, 2008).

Criterion 5: Recurrent suicidal behavior, gestures or threats, or self-mutilating behavior

Self-harm refers to harm inflicted upon the body, usually as a means of relieving emotional distress, and can take many forms, including overdosing, cutting, hitting, scratching, burning, pulling hair, and deliberately getting beaten up. Self-harm and suicidal behaviors serve the function of decreasing emotional distress either directly or indirectly by encouraging people in the environment to respond in a manner that decreases the person's short-term distress. Not infrequently, the idea of suicide and/or suicide planning can result in the person feeling less distressed, having an awareness of suicide as a back-up (albeit highly dysfunctional) solution to their distress. The dangers of this process are obvious and serious.

Criterion 6: Affective instability due to a marked reactivity of mood (e.g., intense episodic dysphoria, irritability or anxiety usually lasting a few hours and only rarely more than a few days)

Do your client's emotions shift rapidly and unpredictably in response to internal or external cues or sometimes for reasons that the person has yet to identify? This may seem like an intense roller-coaster ride, with the person feeling out of control of their emotions and actions, and that instead their emotions are controlling them. Because emotions are so intense and labile, it is more challenging to use skilful ways of coping when distressed. It is more likely therefore that your client's behavior will be determined by their mood; that is, mood-dependent actions and responses dominate rather than skilful behaviors and reflection, whatever their mood.

Consumer comment

I experienced extremely intense and floridly raging emotions. When these emotions were distressing, all my actions were driven towards avoiding feeling as I tried consciously (and now recognize also unconsciously) to completely suppress my experience. When I "succeeded," I felt nothing; a kind of emotional neutrality or numbness. This unfortunately seemed to be only temporarily effective at not feeling, with the feelings often returning with even greater intensity with the next trigger. The result of this was that very little of my actions was wise. Instead it was mood dependant, creating even further problems and distress over time (Jackson, personal communication).

Criterion 7: Chronic feelings of emptiness

Does your client describe a painful feeling of emptiness or hollowness inside? Emptiness has a number of different causes. Understandably, if peoples' lives have involved numerous disappointments they may become fearful of trying things and fearful of engaging in life; they may avoid a lot of things to try decrease their distress. Unfortunately this is likely to leave the person with not enough going on in their life that is meaningful. Shutting out/avoiding emotions will leave people without the ability to know what is meaningful and satisfying, and therefore feeling empty. Attempts to fill this emptiness whilst either avoiding engaging in life or blocking the experience of emotions may be to no avail. This is like trying to fill a bucket with water when the bucket has holes in the base. Emptiness is also likely to result from difficulties establishing and maintaining satisfying intimate attached relationships that would otherwise be fulfilling and give a person a sense of recognition and completeness.

Consumer comment

It was not until I read the diagnostic criteria for BPD that I was able to put words to the big hole inside me. I felt that I was hollow and worthless, and that my existence had no meaning or substance. Later, I needed to be constantly active to fill the black hole in me (Krawitz & Jackson, 2008).

Criterion 8: Inappropriate intense anger or difficulty controlling anger (e.g., frequent displays of temper, constant anger, recurrent physical fights)

Is your client easily cued into rages? Anger may be experienced by all of us in response to our experience of frustrated needs and experience of disappointment and can be a very powerful experience that may be overwhelming. Being angry in itself is not necessarily a problem. DSM uses the language of "inappropriate" here to refer to anger leading to actions (such as assault) that are contrary to the person's best interests or outside socially recognized norms and are so excessive that viable relationships become impossible. People with BPD might be biologically primed to experience emotions intensely, including the emotion of anger. Also, if their worldview is that important people should be perfect then it will be inevitable that rage will occur when this unrealistic expectation is not met.

Criterion 9: Transient, stress-related paranoid ideation or severe dissociative symptoms

If our clients have had past experiences of feeling misunderstood by people, or worse that people have been dangerous (e.g., physical/or sexual assault), it is likely that they will be supersensitive to and highly watchful for danger. This can sometimes result in an over-reaction to incorrectly perceived danger, when none exists. This may result in wariness or even frank paranoid thinking.

Your client may be someone who intentionally or unintentionally dissociates as a way of not feeling. Dissociation may take milder forms of detachment—"feeling numb" or "switching out," where the person is simultaneously aware of dissociating—or more extreme forms where the person has no awareness of dissociating and has memory absences for event/s and periods of time.

Consumer comment

At times of stress I have had experiences of completely "losing time," becoming aware of being in a different place (even city) to where I last recalled and having no idea of the time or day. Whilst I have been able to "choose" to dissociate, 90% of the time the experience has come upon me without choosing (Jackson, personal communication).

Dissociation and self-harm as discriminating features

Severe dissociation (Zanarini, Ruser, Frankenberg, & Hennen, 2000) and persistent self-harm correlate with a diagnosis of BPD and are probably the two most discriminating features in making a diagnosis. Of course, neither self-harm nor severe dissociation is sufficient for the diagnosis. Many people who do not meet criteria for BPD self-harm or severely dissociate. The literature is less clear about what percentage of people who engage in an episode of self-harm meet diagnostic criteria for BPD, as most studies of suicidal behavior have not reported on Axis II diagnoses (Linehan, 1993a). See sections on co-occurring conditions and understanding self-harm later in this chapter for further information.

Understanding borderline personality disorder

It is important to recognize that the diagnosis of BPD is only one part of understanding the unique personhood of the individual with BPD and that the diagnosis is integrated with other ways of understanding the person. Identification of specific and unique factors that maintain problems will guide personalized, validating, and humanizing treatment planning and suggest solutions specific to our clients.

Consumer comment

When I was diagnosed with BPD, the common language used was that I "was" a borderline personality disorder. I hated this, emphasizing for me the sense that I was entirely damaged. As consumers we speak of ourselves as "someone who meets diagnostic criteria for BPD" or as someone "who has BPD." This sits much better with me, as it indicates that this is just one part of what made up the person that was me (Krawitz & Jackson, 2008).

Grouping DSM-IV-TR diagnostic criteria

One way of thinking about the main features of BPD is to group the DSM-IV-TR diagnostic criteria into three groupings:

- *emotion group* (highly reactive mood and emotions, unstable relationships, emptiness, abandonment fears, intense anger)
- *impulsivity group* (e.g., self-harm, substance use)
- *identity group* (emptiness, abandonment fears, unstable self-image/sense of self).

Many people consider adding a sensitivity group (paranoid thinking) as some patients' main symptoms may be related to a self-referent and crippling interpretation of the world and a sensitivity to others' views of them.

Linehan's biological vulnerability theory

Linehan's (1993a) theory is that people with BPD might have a constitutional biological vulnerability that predisposes them to developing BPD. This biological vulnerability comprises:

- high sensitivity (low threshold of emotional response to situations)
- high reactivity (emotional response is large)
- slow return to baseline (emotional distress persists over time).

This biological emotional sensitivity and intensity is neither good nor bad and has advantages and disadvantages that can be worked with.

Emotional sensitivity

There is now some research evidence that people with BPD have high baseline emotion sensitivity, especially to unpleasant emotions (Jacob et al., 2008, 2009; Kuo & Linehan, 2009; Rosenthal, Gratz, Cheavens, Lejuez, & Lynch, 2008). This research is congruent with clinical experience, where a number of people with BPD and clinicians have described the emotional sensitivity of people with BPD as being like that of the physical sensitivity of people with severe extensive burns. One of us (Roy) worked for a few months many years ago in a hospital burns unit. The physical pain of the patients was enormous, as can no doubt be imagined. The burns left people with understandable skin sensitivity, where what would have been for others slight changes, such as movement of the sheets, caused pain of a level that words seemed unable to communicate. Another simile is that the emotional intensity and distress of people with BPD is a bit like the pain of being romantically dumped, which some of us might have experienced, except that the pain does not lessen with the passage of time (with the permission of Ruth E.S. Allen).

Consumer comment

It seemed that behaviors that appeared insignificant to others could lead to emotional reactions from me of stratospheric proportions. It seemed that no action, including severe self-harm, or words could effectively communicate to others the intensity of my experience. Other people didn't seem to "get it," not that I made it easy for them. Caring meaningful attempts at expressions of empathy by others led to derision from me as I did not believe that anyone could possibly understand the intensity of my pain.

Even when the seemingly insignificance or "smallness" of the trigger was apparent to me on an intellectual level, I struggled to express to anyone how I could be upset by such an apparently insignificant comment, action or inaction (Jackson, personal communication).

Mentalizing vulnerability

Fonagy and others have proposed that people with BPD have a vulnerability to losing mentalizing abilities, particularly in interpersonal interactions. (Fonagy & Bateman, 2008a; Fonagy, Gergely, Jurist, Elliot, & Target 2002; Fonagy, Target, & Gergely, 2000). This vulnerability arises from a complex interaction between temperamental and developmental factors. People with BPD are left with a biology of "being frazzled" and easily taken "off-line" (Arnsten, 1998). People with BPD are uniquely sensitive to interpersonal stress and the brain "brakes" in the higher brain centers fail to control the "gas pedal" located in the lower centers. The model takes into account constitutional vulnerability and is rooted in attachment theory and its elaboration by contemporary developmental psychologists (Fonagy, 2003; Fonagy & Bateman, 2007, 2008b; Gergely, 2001). The model suggests that disruption of the attachment relationship early in development in combination with later traumatic experiences in an attachment context interacts with neurobiological development. The combination leads to hyper-responsiveness of the attachment system, which makes mentalizing, the capacity to make sense of ourselves and others in terms of mental states, unstable during emotional arousal. The emergence of earlier modes of psychological function at these times accounts for the symptoms of BPD such as:

+ frantic efforts to avoid abandonment
+ pattern of unstable and intense interpersonal relationships
+ rapidly escalating tempo moving from acquaintance to great intimacy
+ emotional dyscontrol.

Beck's core schemas

"Schemas are core beliefs that act as templates or underlying rules for information processing" and function to "screen, filter, code and assign information from the environment." (Wright, Basco, & Thase, 2006)

Beck et al. (1990) describe people with BPD as often having three core schemas:

+ the world is dangerous and malevolent
+ I am powerless and vulnerable
+ I am inherently unacceptable

and describes how these core schemas might interface:

Some persons who view the world as a dangerous, malevolent place believe that they can rely on their own strengths and abilities in dealing with the threats it presents. However, borderline individuals' belief that they are weak and powerless blocks this solution. Other individuals who believe that they are not capable of dealing effectively with the demands of daily life resolve their dilemma by becoming dependent on someone who they see as capable of taking care of them (and develop a dependent pattern). However, borderlines' belief that they are inherently unacceptable blocks this solution, since this belief leads them to conclude that dependence entails a serious risk of rejection, abandonment, or attack if this inherent unacceptability is discovered. Borderline individuals face quite a dilemma: convinced that they are relatively helpless in a hostile world but without a source of security, they are forced to vacillate between autonomy and dependence without being able to rely on either (Beck & Freeman, 1990).

Reproduced from Beck, A.T., Freeman, A., Cognitive therapy of
personality disorders © 1990, Guilford Press, with permission.

Dichotomous/all or nothing thinking

Dichotomous/all or nothing (black and white) thinking is common in people with BPD and has been illuminated to some degree in our discussion on DSM-IV-TR diagnostic criteria. If our clients feel that life is like a roller-coaster ride, this is one of the primary reasons.

Consumer comment

I have decided that all or nothing thinking is not "all" in people with BPD and "nothing" in others, being not that uncommon in the general population, just not so extreme. Having got that need of mine to normalize at least part of my experience off my chest, so to speak, it is a real issue that I have struggled to decrease as I have healed. However, I can now recognize this thinking and challenge myself as it is happening; laugh compassionately at/with myself and quietly remind myself of the value of recognizing multiple perspectives and truths. This has certainly enhanced my capacity to make and maintain relationships (Jackson, personal communication).

Strong sense of justice—aiming for justice at the expense of being effective

Many people with BPD are sensitized to injustice because of the injustices of their past experiences, with a fierce determination for justice to prevail in all circumstances. Both justice and looking after oneself are important. There are significant disadvantages in idealistically "going down in a blaze of bullets" for a cause that does not justify the risks our clients may be placing themselves in. It is important that our clients live to "fight another day" and that for them "winning the battle" is less important than winning the struggle to recovery.

Harsh on self (and others)

Perhaps related to seeing the world in absolute all-or-nothing ways is the anger our clients might feel for themselves and others when their expectations are not met. We have not met any single group of people who are consistently harder on themselves than people with BPD. This is a very sad irony. Many people with BPD have had very difficult pasts and are in need of a high level of self-acceptance. If the world were a fair place and justice prevailed, then people with BPD would, because of their difficult pasts, have a view of themselves that was compassionate, caring, and accepting. Unfortunately often quite the opposite occurs, as people with BPD often internalize the invalidating or critical messages about themselves that might have been given. This then results in a harsh view of themselves and sometimes others.

Consumer comment

I have had no harsher critic than myself. When I lived with the turmoil of BPD I hated myself for being unable live up to my own high expectations, let alone anyone else's. This led to me isolating myself and not engaging in life to avoid failing by not meeting my extreme standards. This led to further self-hatred and an increased sense of isolation and desperation— further reminding me of how useless I was. These days I can consciously remind myself that I am an OK person even if not perfect or the very best at everything I do—something I was unable to do in the past (Jackson, personal communication).

Fluctuating competence

Some people with BPD can have times of high levels of competence only to rapidly decompensate following a prompting event, whether identifiable or not, into a low level of competence. Some are competent in certain situations but unable to sustain this competence in other situations. This can be very difficult for our clients and others, and once again can be part of the roller-coaster ride of extreme ups and downs. Family and friends may also be perplexed by this rapid change from competence to incompetence. It can also be disconcerting for strangers who are stunned by our clients' sudden deterioration in competence.

Consumer comment

For a part of my recovery I was able to be incredibly functional in a work situation, but struggled immensely at the end of each working day. It was almost like I used all my resources up while at work and had none left when I was outside work. This was really hard to understand for me and others. Many of my work colleagues could not understand how they saw a competent and capable person at work who was desperate and needing high levels of support outside of work. I often felt that they thought I was deliberately not coping at certain times of day. The fact was, that with the clear expectations, goals and support in my working day, I well understood what was required of me, and how to "be" or behave, and knew I was capable in that situation. I had none of those structures or supports in my personal life, and so could not manage my nonwork life (Krawitz & Jackson, 2008).

Active passivity

Active passivity is a term used by Linehan (1993a,b), referring to a situation where a person actively works hard on being passive.

An example might include telling another person about a problem that they have and actively encouraging the other person to fix the problem or passively waiting for them to fix it. If our clients have not built a history of success doing things, they might feel demoralized and helpless about their capacity to ever be successful at doing things for themselves. It then makes sense that our clients will try to get others to do things for them. The desire to avoid what is perceived of as yet another inevitable failure can understandably result in our clients being very active in ensuring they are passive. This style can be effective at times in getting other people to do things for our clients, but if this is our clients' dominant style it has the major downside of making sure they will

CO-OCCURRING CONDITIONS | **19**

not be learning life skills and may interfere with developing and maintaining functional relationships. There are clear dangers that need to be addressed where this active passivity includes our clients' approach to their therapy and recovery.

Consumer comment

I know that people perceived me as being "actively passive" and seemed to think this was deliberate. The fact was, I did not believe I had the power to change, and the only way I could see myself getting out of any situation that I was in, was for the situation to be changed by someone else, or for someone to remove or protect me from the situation (Krawitz & Jackson, 2008).

Co-occurring conditions

Considering the enduring and pervasive difficulties and distress that our clients with BPD experience it is not the least bit surprising that they will frequently get depressed or anxious or use a variety of means such as self-harm, substances, gambling, and restricted and binge eating to deal with their distress, which will result in meeting the criteria for other co-occurring conditions. It is only a minority of people with BPD who have "pure" BPD with no other diagnoses. Stone's (1989) study of people with BPD found only 37% had a "pure" diagnosis of BPD, with no co-occurring diagnosis, and this study took place at a private US facility. It is likely that those with multiple co-occurring conditions will be those that present the greatest challenges to services.

We list here some of the more common co-occurring DSM-IV-TR Axis I diagnoses associated with BPD in people with BPD, across a range of different studies (Krawitz & Watson, 2003; Zanarini, Frankenburg, Hennen, Bradford Reich, & Silk, 2004; Korzekwa, Dell, Links, Thabane, & Fougere, 2009):

- major depressive disorder (35–85%)
- dysthymic disorder (25–65%)
- bipolar affective disorder (uncertain, perhaps 1–15%)
- generalized anxiety disorder (10%)
- panic disorder (30–50%)
- agoraphobia (10–35%)
- social phobia (25–50%)
- post-traumatic stress disorder (35–55%)
- obsessive–compulsive disorder (15–25%)

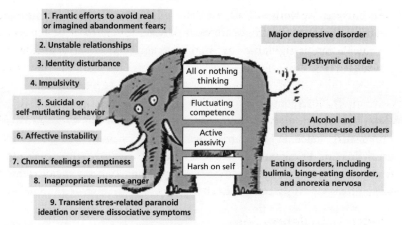

Fig. 1.1 Understanding BPD: BPD DSM-IV-TR criteria reworded[1-9] and co-occurring diagnoses or problems associated with BPD. Adapted from and printed with the permission of Kiera Van Gelder, President, Middle Path, consumer organization dedicated to the advocacy, support and education of those affected by BPD (Kiera van Gelder's figure in turn was inspired by something similar from Valerie Porr).

- ◆ alcohol and other substance dependence or abuse (20–65%)
- ◆ bulimia (25–40%)
- ◆ binge-eating disorder
- ◆ eating disorder (any eating disorder—30–50%)
- ◆ dissociation (mild to severe—76%)
- ◆ attention deficit hyperactivity disorder (16–38%).

Figure 1.1 is an adaptation from a colleague (Kiera van Gelder, inspired by something similar from Valerie Porr) who has used the parable of the elephant to illustrate various features of BPD. In the parable a number of blind people touching an elephant described the elephant completely differently. One person holding a tusk described the elephant as a plough, another holding a foot as a pillar, and another holding the tail as a brush. It is the same with BPD. Up close we may see some parts in great detail but not others and need to step back to be able to see all of what the BPD condition may involve. On the left-hand side is what we think is the concise core of the DSM-IV-TR features of BPD; on the right-hand side are common co-occurring conditions and in the centre some of the ways of understanding BPD described earlier.

Suicide

Thoughts of suicide are very common in people with BPD. Often these thoughts are around for quite a long time with periods of greater and lesser intensity.

The clients that we work with almost universally have had a daily background level of suicidal thoughts that are intensified in response to specific situations. The suicide rate is significant, with older studies suggesting a suicide rate of 10% (Paris & Zweig-Frank, 2001; Stone, 1990) over a 25-year follow-up, a rate 50 times higher than the general population (American Psychiatric Association, 2001). Zanarini et al's (Zanarini, Frankenburg, Hennen, Reich, & Silk) more recent study had a 4% suicide rate at 10-year follow-up (Zanarini, Frankenburg, Reich, & Fitzmaurice, 2010a)and 4.5% at 16-year follow-up to date (Zanarini, Frankenburg, Reich, & Fitzmaurice, 2012). As newer more effective treatments are being provided, it is plausible that the suicide rate will lessen. This is certainly our anecdotal experience.

Overlap with depression

There is a considerable relationship between BPD and depressive disorder, and BPD and dysthymic disorder that is vigorously debated but not yet completely resolved (Gunderson et al., 2004). At a treatment level it will not be surprising if our clients are depressed or dysthymic, given their difficult past and current life problems.

Overlap with bipolar disorder

There is overlap between the symptoms of BPD and bipolar affective disorder, the nature of which is not yet resolved (Gunderson et al., 2004; Magill, 2004; Stone, 2006). When the differential diagnosis includes BPD and bipolar affective disorder, accurate diagnosis where possible will greatly improve outcome. Accurate diagnosis of bipolar disorder will usually mean that medication treatment will have a major role in treatment planning. Accurate diagnosis of BPD, on the other hand, will lead to a somewhat different treatment plan where therapy is the dominant treatment. The presenting symptoms of BPD can be remarkably similar to those of a brittle, rapidly fluctuating form of bipolar disorder. Compared to people with bipolar disorder, people with BPD have emotional shifts which tend to be of shorter duration, of more rapid onset and termination, and more immediately linked to an identifiable environmental stressor, often with a strong interpersonal context. Sometimes BPD and bipolar affective disorder occur together, probably at a rate higher than one would expect in the general population.

Interface with psychotic phenomena

The interface between psychotic experiences and BPD has also generated considerable debate and again the area remains somewhat unresolved. Research suggests that psychotic symptoms that do not attract a diagnosis of schizophrenia or bipolar affective disorder are more common in post-traumatic stress disorder (Chan & Silove, 2000; Hamner, Frueh, Ulmer, & Arana, 1999; Ivezic, Oruc, & Bell, 1999; Sautter et al., 1999; Umgvari & Mullen, 2000). The presence of psychotic symptoms, whilst inviting consideration of a diagnosis of schizophrenia or bipolar disorder, is not sufficient for the diagnosis. Transient paranoid thinking is one of the DSM-IV-TR diagnostic criteria for BPD. The presence of auditory hallucinosis (hallucination where the person knows that the auditory perception originates from themselves and not externally; often referred phenomenologically loosely in the context of BPD as "borderline voices"; Yee, Korner, McSwiggan, Meares, & Stevenson, 2005)) and brief psychotic episodes are not unusual in people meeting diagnostic criteria for BPD without the person meeting any of the other diagnostic criteria for schizophrenia or bipolar affective disorder.

Interface with dissociation

Dissociation may be milder or more severe and may include the following phenomena: experience of disconnection with emotion, numbness, going blank, derealization (out-of-body experiences), depersonalization (outside of self experiences), some "flashback" experiences (believing or feeling as if one is in the past trauma situation), amnesic periods, and experience of separate identities.

Korzekwa et al. (2009) report studies demonstrating dissociative identity disorder to occur in 10–27% of people with BPD and for BPD to occur in 30–70% of people with dissociative identity disorder. In their sample of 21 people with BPD, Korzekwa et al. (2009) found 76% to have dissociative symptoms stating that "the average BPD patient endorsed a wide variety of deeply disturbing dissociative symptoms that were anything but "transient and stress related,"" arguing for greater consideration to be given to dissociation symptoms in DSM criteria.

Overlap with other personality disorders

BPD is one of 11 personality disorder categories defined in DSM-IV-TR. If our client meets diagnostic criteria for BPD there is a good chance they will meet diagnostic criteria for another personality disorder/s. This is not meant to alarm but highlights the fact that the personality disorder categories often overlap significantly.

The more commonly associated personality disorders and prevalence in BPD (Zanarini et al., 1998; Zanarini, Frankenburg, Hennen, Reich, & Silk, 2004) are:

- avoidant personality disorder (35–45%)
- dependent personality disorder (40–50%)

- paranoid personality disorder (20–30%)
- antisocial personality disorder (15–25%; likely to be higher in forensic and prison services).

It is not in the least surprising that avoidant, dependent, and paranoid personality disorder are associated with BPD as these are perfectly understandable responses to difficult pasts. If our clients have been unsuccessful in past activities, avoiding situations is an understandable way of coping with high anxiety, albeit problematic, which if extensive could manifest with behaviors of someone with avoidant personality disorder. If our clients have low self-confidence it makes sense, albeit problematic, that they will look to others for solutions to life's problems, which if pervasive could manifest with behaviors of someone with dependent personality disorder. If our clients have not been understood or have been abused by others it is understandable that they will be wary of people which, if full blown, could manifest with behaviors of someone with paranoid personality disorder.

There is some overlap between BPD and antisocial personality disorder. A pervasive failure of empathy is not a criterion in the DSM-IV-TR diagnosis of antisocial personality disorder, but it was a clinically meaningful part of the old diagnostic terminology of psychopathy. People meeting diagnostic criteria for BPD frequently may have antisocial traits, but are able to be empathic to another's experience, sometimes exquisitely so, at least for short periods. People meeting diagnostic criteria for BPD clearly have empathic capacity, often to a considerable degree, although it is not usually sustained and consistent, and may occur only when things are going well.

Etiology

Biological factors

Research has shown that people with BPD are statistically more likely to have altered brain anatomy and functioning, including smaller volumes of the amygdala and hippocampus (Nunes et al., 2009), a "sluggish serotonin system" (Gurvitz, Koenigsberg, & Siever, 2000), and abnormal brain electrical activity (Boutros, Torello, & McGlashan, 2003). Sluggish serotonin systems are statistically associated with lowered mood, depression, irritability, anger, and impulsivity. Porr uses the metaphors of the amygdala being the brain's emotional gas pedal (overactive in BPD), the pre-frontal cortex being the brain's emotional brake (underactive in BPD), and serotonin being the brain system's oil (Porr, 2010). It is not yet known whether these physiological and anatomical brain differences are a predisposition to developing BPD, a response to life experiences or some combination of these two factors.

There is some evidence that people with BPD have a biological higher intensity of emotional experiencing, particularly of displeasing emotions (Jacob et al., 2008; Rosenthal et al., 2008; Kuo & Linehan, 2009). As mentioned earlier, dialectical behavior therapy (DBT) hypothesizes that some people with BPD may be born with a biological predisposition of emotion intensity and sensitivity. Parents of children with BPD describe problems as early as infancy compared to their other children or other children that they know who did not develop BPD (Goodman et al., 2010). Emotion intensity and sensitivity are neither good nor bad and both have advantages and disadvantages. However, if parents themselves do not experience emotions as intensely, it will understandably be difficult for them to know what the experience of emotional intensity is like and they will not have had the personal experience of successfully making the most out of this temperament. It would be hard for any parent in this circumstance to model how to deal with intense emotions or how to teach their child to work with their intense emotions. The quality of the parenting received may have been sufficient for other children born less sensitive but was unfortunately insufficient for the person, born emotionally sensitive. So, the sad situation here is that even the most caring of parents may be unable to teach their child how to work with manage and celebrate their intense emotions. If this happens, the child may feel misunderstood, which will then impact on the parents, who may feel unappreciated, ineffective at parenting, and misunderstood, and a cycle of misunderstanding may become embedded. This understanding might assist the person with BPD and their family to move beyond blame towards solutions.

It is increasingly recognized that there is a substantial genetic contribution to personality. Data from twin studies demonstrates genetic contributions to BPD of 30–50% (Bornovalova, Hicks, Iacono, & McGue, 2009; Distel et al., 2008), with Distel et al.'s study demonstrating the same genetic contributions (42%) across three countries (The Netherlands, Belgium, Australia). Genetic factors may manifest as personality traits such as emotion intensity, sensitivity and reactivity, impulsivity, irritability, and novelty-seeking. One large study (Torgersen et al., 2000) of identical and nonidentical twins of people with BPD showed that the identical twins had a five times increased chance of having BPD compared to nonidentical twins. (A much smaller earlier twin study did not demonstrate a likelihood of BPD being inherited, possibly due to the small study size.)

Another study of people diagnosed with a depressive disorder showed that 8% of people without a particular gene and without a history of childhood sexual abuse had a history of having self-harmed. This rose to 30–36% where either the gene was present or there was a history of childhood sexual abuse, and to 60% where both the gene was present and there was a history of childhood sexual abuse (Joyce et al., 2006). The conclusions of this study are that both biological and psychological factors contribute to self-harm which is most frequent when both biological and psychological factors exist.

Psychological factors

Widom et al. (2009) report an increased risk of BPD 30 years later in a prospective study of children with court-documented physical abuse or neglect. Zanarini et al. (1997) document 92% of clients retrospectively reporting childhood neglect, 59% childhood physical abuse, and 29% prolonged childhood separation. Retrospective histories of sexual abuse are reported by about 70% of clients by Laporte and Guttman (1996) and Zanarini et al. (1997). Whilst sexual abuse is correlated with a diagnosis of BPD, it is neither necessary (30–70% have no abuse history) nor sufficient (the vast majority of people who are sexually abused do not develop BPD). Being brought up in an environment that was abusive or neglectful will obviously have a profound impact on our psychological development, decreasing our chances of entering adulthood with secure attachments, psychological skills, good self-esteem, and confidence.

Nature and nurture—interplay of biological and psychological factors

Most international experts are in agreement that biological and psychological factors can contribute to the development of the condition and that there is often interplay between these biological and psychological factors. However, there is dispute regarding the relative contributions of these two factors. A large amount of information now exists that the debate of nature versus nurture is dated and has been replaced with "nature and nurture, nature via nurture or nurture via nature."

Sociocultural factors

Sociocultural factors may protect or predispose to developing BPD. Risk factors might include changed and changing social roles and expectations, loss of the extended family, societal breakdown, and substance use cultures. Protective factors might include a connected intact society, clear role expectations, extended family networks, and cultures that place high value on interpersonal attachment and connection.

Unique set of multiple interacting factors

The pathway to developing the disorder will be unique for each of our clients with different predisposing or protecting factors from biological, psychological, and sociocultural sources. For example, some people will have had a high genetic predisposition and require only a small environmental contribution to push past the threshold for having BPD. On the other hand, another person may have had little genetic predisposing factors but had such devastating trauma (such as repeated ongoing childhood sexual abuse from an early age) that this was sufficient to push through the threshold. If the sexual abuse occurred as a child, how people that our clients shared this with responded could have been predisposing or protective. A validating response where people were believing, supportive, and ensured that the abuse never happened again would have been somewhat protective compared to a severely invalidating response where our clients were not believed, not supported, and not protected from further abuse.

An etiological pathway that might apply to your client could have a starting point of being born with predisposing physiology such as high emotional experiencing and/or childhood emotional trauma. As a consequence of either or both of these factors, relationships were affected, and physiology and possibly brain "hard wiring" altered, decreasing secure attachments, learning capacity and increasing impulsivity, emotional instability and sensitivity to stress. This, in turn, impacted on relationships, which in turn affected brain function and so on. High sensitivity and reactivity to emotional events, unstable emotions, identity problems, relationship problems, poor self-image, and counterproductive self-talk resulted; in time the behaviors and internal experiences of someone meeting diagnostic criteria for BPD developed.

Why are more females diagnosed with BPD?

A US national epidemiological community study of 35,000 people showed no gender difference in prevalence rates (Grant et al., 2008). This study needs replication. However, assuming its accuracy requires some hypotheses as to why more females are diagnosed with BPD than males, which include:

- males with psychological problems seek out professional help less frequently
- males with the same behaviors more likely to receive a diagnosis of antisocial personality disorder
- males may be more likely to be found in substance use, justice services and anti-violence programs where the diagnosis of BPD is made less frequently. A significant percentage of perpetrators of family violence (who are more frequently male) might meet diagnostic criteria for BPD.

Understanding self-harm

The definition of self-harm that we use in this book is: an action intended to do physical harm to the body without intending to die, which serves a short-term function.

Self-harm behaviors include (but are not limited to):

- taking too many tablets/overdosing
- swallowing poisons/caustic substances
- cutting
- scratching skin
- burning (e.g., with cigarettes)
- banging head
- hitting/punching self
- throwing body against something
- starting confrontation, so as to be physically beaten
- jumping from height
- pulling hair out
- preventing wounds from healing
- making medical situations worse (e.g., not taking insulin as prescribed)
- applying poisons/caustic substances on skin
- stabbing/puncturing self
- sticking things into body (e.g., vagina, urethra)
- swallowing objects.

The most common forms of self-harm in people with BPD in mental health settings are overdosing and cutting. Behaviors such as alcohol, drug use, cigarette smoking, binge eating, and sex with strangers may have very similar functions to self-harm and be equally dangerous, but are not usually subsumed under the label of "self-harm" unless the intentional purpose of these behaviors is to harm the body.

There is no single cause and there are very individual reasons as to why people self-harm. We do know that self-harm can rapidly bring back a feeling of being in control, reduce tension, and relieve unbearable anguish and so easily becomes a "quick fix" for inner turmoil. The function of self-harm in people with BPD is almost always to decrease distress, and can be categorized as decreasing distress directly or decreasing distress indirectly by effects on people in the environment.

Patients deal with internal distress directly in order to:

- "feel better"
- change emotional pain into physical pain
- make "invisible" emotional pain visible
- distract
- deal with high anxiety
- deal with high levels of anger
- punish oneself
- feel something
- feel alive
- not feel, feel numb or dissociate
- prevent feeling numb or dissociated
- feel grounded or whole
- feel in control
- care for oneself (look after wound caringly).

In these situations, self-harm is a private action and accounts for the large majority of self-harm behaviors. The purpose of the self-harm is achieved without anybody having to know about the self-harm.

Consumer comment

Initially, when I started self-harming the sole intention was to distract from the intense distressing emotions I was feeling and to regain a sense of control. My self-harm was very measured and "controlled" to ensure I stopped just short of requiring medical intervention so that no other person would know I was self-harming. (Jackson, personal communication)

In contrast to dealing with distress directly through self-harm, patients may deal with internal distress indirectly, that is, via the signal the action gives to others. Self-harm is used to:

- communicate to others
- communicate intensity of distress to others
- feel heard
- attract caring responses from others
- get access to mental health services

- control others
- punish others.

In these situations, self-harm is a public action and accounts for a minority of self-harm behaviors, although they are often the ones that generate high clinician concern. The purpose of the self-harm can only be achieved if others know about the self-harm.

Consumer comment

Whilst my initial self-harming was a deliberately private act intended to privately alleviate my suffering, I quickly discovered my incredible need, or perceived need, to be cared for and helped would be met by professionals if I self-harmed, or threatened to self-harm. (Jackson, personal communication)

Some clients may express the idea that if self-harm works to reduce distress, why stop? Clinicians need to be ready to respond to this question, possibly as follows. Self-harm has a high correlation with suicide, and whilst this could be a severity correlation, it is also very likely that self-harm behaviors prime the person psychologically and possibly neurobiologically to suicide. That is, it is a small step to move from self-harm as a means of dealing with distress to suicide as a means of dealing with distress. Self-harm behaviors as a means of dealing with distress also critically prevent our clients learning and practicing alternative effective ways of dealing with life situations, which is what is required for our clients to reduce their future risk of suicide.

Everyone who self-harms should be taken seriously and the events discussed.

Prognosis

Do people with BPD get better or recover? An emphatic yes! People with BPD do generally get better and recover.

What recovery means will be different for each person. For some it may be a decrease in distressing symptoms to the point where life is worth living on more days than earlier. For others it may be feeling that life is worth living on more days than not. For many people it is much more than this.

Zanarini et al. (Zanarini, Frankenburg, Hennen, & Silk, 2003) in a naturalistic study followed up people initially hospitalized in the USA (50% recipients of government health insurance). At 8-year follow-up 68% and at 10-year follow-up 86% of people initially diagnosed with BPD had had a sustained remission (had not met diagnostic criteria for more than 4 years) (Zanarini et al., 2006, 2008, 2010a, 2011; Zanarini, Frankenburg, Hennen, Bradford Reich, et al., 2004). Relapse rates were low compared with other major psychiatric conditions such as mood disorders and schizophrenia, with a 33% relapse rate in the 8 years following going into remission. These results are far more optimistic than views on prognosis a few decades ago. Psychosocial functioning at 10-year follow-up, as categorized by Zanarini et al. (2010a), demonstrated 78% with "Good psychosocial function broadly defined," 64% with "Good psychosocial function narrowly defined," and 50% defined as diagnostically and psychosocially "recovered." The definitions used were as follows:

"Good psychosocial function broadly defined": One sustaining committed relationship (close weekly contact without abuse or neglect) with a friend or romantic partner + good sustained vocational performance and history (vocation—work, study, parenting, stay-at-home houseperson).

"Good psychosocial function narrowly defined": Above + full-time vocation history

"Recovered": Above + in remission for more than 4 years. Social functioning was far more stable and much more achievable than vocational functioning, with vocational deficits accounting for the overwhelming majority of poor psychosocial functioning. This appears to become a long-term problem. Vocational deficits continue at 16 years follow-up (Zanarini et al., 2012). Clinical implications of this might be that treatments need to place increased attention on vocational skills and rehabilitation models, and offer treatment intermittently over the long term (Bateman, 2012).

Does time heal?

Earlier studies following people for a long period of time show that people do improve with the passage of time (Paris & Zweig-Frank, 2001; Stone, 1990). Researchers believe that this was not just a direct result of treatment but also a feature of time specifically. Improvement over time is thought to be related to both biological changes over time that result in decreased impulsivity and also to gradual learning of psychological skills over time.

Consumer comment

When I was diagnosed with BPD, my first reaction was one of hopelessness—my prior knowledge was that there was no effective treatment—for a long time there was no research indicating otherwise. Fortunately I was lucky enough to have some wonderful clinicians who fully believed in my ability to get better—mostly they believed more than I did, and often it was only their belief in my ability to have a life that kept me going. The really exciting thing is that their belief in my ability to recover was not a false hope, and now there is research available to confirm this. It is likely that with modern treatments your clients will get better—the research says so!! (Krawitz & Jackson, 2008)

Psychosocial treatment outcome studies

Generalist treatments

The growing evidence of the effectiveness of high-quality generalist treatment for BPD led to the writing of this book and this evidence is the subject of more detailed discussion in Chapter 2.

Specialist treatments

The first randomized controlled trial of the effectiveness of psychotherapy for BPD was published in 1991, with nearly 20 randomized controlled trials published subsequently. Evidence is now unequivocal that psychological treatments for people with BPD are effective. The naturalistic prognosis studies are hopeful in that we can reasonably expect that people with BPD will improve over time. If your clients are engaged in evidence-based therapy/ies, then it is likely that they will on balance recover quicker and probably with a greater robustness to their recovery. It is exciting that there are now a number of psychological treatments that have evidence of effectiveness. As a profession this increases our and our clients' options to best match client, clinician, resources, and treatment model. Some clients who do not respond to one evidence-based treatment might respond to another evidence-based treatment. The numbers of studies published are increasing and we can look forward to an ever growing evidence of psychotherapy treatment effectiveness.

Expert agreement is that psychotherapy is the primary treatment for BPD with medication to assist, and that treatment is longer-term. All the stand-alone treatments in the research have been for a minimum of 12 months with treatment duration limited by research rather than clinical criteria.

If your client has had years of treatment without improvement, do not give up. Research has shown that change in many areas of human endeavor may take several attempts before being successful at another attempt. This is well recognized in the area of addictions, where people addicted to nicotine, alcohol or heroin have successfully changed their behaviors and stopped smoking, using alcohol or using heroin after previous unsuccessful efforts. If your client has had unsuccessful previous treatment/s, assess what you both can do this time around that will increase the likelihood of recovery. Whilst severity is understandably a poorer prognostic indicator, there is also a silver lining to this in that there is research on the STEPPS (systems training for emotional predictability and problem solving) program showing increasing severity predicting greater sizes of improvement (Black, St John, Pfohl, McCormick, & Blum, 2009).

Twelve randomized controlled trials have been cognitive behavior therapy-based and five randomized controlled trials psychodynamically-based for adults with BPD and one randomized controlled trial of cognitive analytic therapy for adolescents with BPD traits. Interestingly the differentiation of treatments into these categories is questionable due to the large overlap between them. DBT is considered by some to be significantly different from CBT and schema focused therapy is more allied to dynamic therapy in its use of the relationship between patient and clinician during treatment.

CBT-based evidence-based treatments

DBT—Nine randomized controlled trials in four centers in North America and Europe (Koons et al., 2001; Linehan, Armstrong, Suarez, Allmon, & Heard, 1991; Linehan et al., 1999, 2002, 2006; McMain, Guimond, Cardish, Streiner, & Links, 2012; McMain et al., 2009; Turner, 2000; Van den Bosch, Koeter, Stijnen, Verhuel, & van den Brink, 2005; Van den Bosch, Verhuel, Schippers, & van den Brink, 2002; Verheul et al., 2003).

STEPPS, a 20-week skills-based group that is an add-on to existing treatment—Two randomized controlled trials in two centers in North America and Europe (Blum et al., 2008; Bos, van Wel, Appelo, & Verbraak, 2010).

Schema-focused therapy—One randomized controlled trial (Gieson-Bloo et al., 2006).

Psychodynamically based evidence-based treatments

Mentalization based therapy—Two randomized controlled trials (Bateman & Fonagy, 1999, 2001, 2003, 2008a, 2009b)

Transference-focused therapy—Two randomized controlled trials in two centers in North America and Europe (Clarkin, Levy, Lenzenweger, & Kernberg, 2007; Doering et al., 2010; Levy et al., 2006).

Relationship management psychodynamic psychotherapy—One randomized controlled trial (Munroe-Blum & Marziali, 1988, 1995).

Cognitive analytic therapy

Cognitive analytic therapy—One randomized controlled trial (Chanen et al., 2008, 2009).

Feasibility

There are also a number of uncontrolled trials that importantly demonstrate the practicality and feasibility of providing effective treatment outside of research settings in "real-world" situations, which is where most BPD treatment takes place (American Psychiatric Association, 1998; Brassington & Krawitz, 2006), one of which, a state-funded community program in New Hampshire, USA, was awarded an American Psychiatric Association Gold Achievement Award for outstanding mental health programs (American Psychiatric Association, 1998).

Pharmacological treatment outcome studies

Pharmacological treatment of BPD is discussed in Chapter 6. Psychotropic medication is effective to a limited degree for different symptoms or dimensions of BPD (NICE, 2009) While there seems to be a shift towards using anti-psychotic and/or mood stabilizers for many of the symptoms of BPD (Abraham & Calabrese, 2008), selective serotonin reuptake inhibitors (SSRIs) remain the most frequently prescribed medication.

Acknowledgements

A substantial amount of the content in this chapter has been adapted from, Krawitz, R., Jackson, W. (2008). Borderline personality disorder: the facts. Oxford: Oxford University Press. The authors wish to thank Wendy Jackson and Oxford University Press for their permission to adapt and use the information from that book for consumers for this book for general mental health clinicians.

Chapter 2

Generalist psychiatric treatments for borderline personality disorder: the evidence base and common factors

Abbreviations used in this chapter only

SCM   a generalist treatment referred to by treatment providers as "structured clinical management"

GPM   a generalist treatment referred to by treatment providers as "general psychiatric management"

GCC   a generalist treatment referred to by treatment developers as "good clinical care"

SP   a generalist treatment referred to by treatment developers as "supportive psychotherapy"

Summary

+ The effectiveness demonstrated in research of the four generalist treatments described in this chapter took the BPD professional world by surprise and was the catalyst for writing this book.

+ Most people with BPD are, and will always be, treated within generalist rather than specialist settings.

+ Generalist treatments are based on skills and knowledge that mostly already exist in the repertoire of reasonably skilled generalist mental health clinicians, thereby requiring relatively modest adaptations rather than learning new techniques, and needing only modest training and supervision to be effective.

- All four of the generalist treatments shown to be effective in research trials show good feasibility and utility, having taken place in real-world clinical contexts and being designed to deliver standardized high-quality treatments that are achievable in economically developed countries.
- Commonalities of the effective generalist treatments that we felt could reasonably be assumed to exist based on the reading of the manuals are the following:

➢ **Initial therapeutic stance**
- Clinicians who choose to work with people with BPD.
- Clinicians who are enthusiastic, hopeful, and welcoming in working with people with BPD.
- Organization willingness.

➢ **Therapy relationship**
- Therapeutic alliance.
- Alliance as
  - treatment goal consensus
  - collaborative agreement on how to achieve these goals.
- Empathy and validation.

➢ **Treatment model features**
- Treatment that is well structured.
- Active clinician to structure interaction.
- Regularity of scheduled sessions as structure for adult treatments.
- Clinician monitoring and quality assurance.
- Treatment model that
  - one believes in
  - has clear focus
  - is theoretically principled and coherent.
- Supervision/team.
- Self-observation—clinician.
- Skills in managing suicidality, including balanced response to suicidality.
- Self-observation—client:
  - identifying emotions
  - analysis of events leading up to and following events, especially sentinel events.

◆ We believe that there will always be important places for both generalist and specialist treatments.

◆ We envisage a hopeful future, where research will guide decision-making at the outset of treatment to best match client severity, stage of change, resources, and other client, clinician, organization, and model characteristics.

In this chapter we:

1. introduce the rationale for seeking common factors in treatment and provide a brief overview of some relevant literature

2. outline the four generalist treatments that have been shown to be effective

3. describe briefly the outcome studies of the four treatments

4. review in more detail commonalities of the treatments

5. provide a table of commonalities across generalist treatments (Table 2.1).

Common features rationale

Most people with BPD are and will always be treated within general mental health services rather than in specialist settings. Generalist treatments are based on skills and knowledge that exist in the repertoire of quality skilled generalist mental health clinicians and require relatively modest adaptations rather than extensive training in new techniques, and only modest levels of continuing supervision to be effective. In discussing the positive outcomes of their generalist treatment, Chanen et al. (2009) state that clinical service reform using existing resources may be more readily achievable and important than the delivery of any specific brand of psychotherapy. International BPD experts (Bateman & Fonagy, 2009b; Paris, 2008; Zanarini, 2009) and ourselves all articulate the need for treatments cheaper than current specialist interventions to be more available and accessible. The 2009 National Institute for Clinical Excellence (NICE) UK government guidelines (NICE, 2009), the 2001 American Psychiatric Association guidelines (American Psychiatric Association, 2001), and the National Health and Medical Research Council Clinical Practice Guideline for the Management of Borderline Personality Disorder in Australia all conclude that high-quality generalist treatments are likely to be "good enough" for most people with BPD. The emphasis here is on "high-quality" generalist treatments that are superior to current standard treatments, which may be ineffective or actually harmful. All the generalist treatments focus on feasibility and utility in real-world clinical

Table 2.1 Commonalities across effective generalist treatments

	SCM	GPM	GCC	SP
Topics discussed in chapter text				
Starting therapeutic stance				
Voluntary, enthusiastic, hopeful and welcoming clinicians	Y	Y	Y	Y
Organization willingness	Y	Y	Y	Y
Therapy relationship				
Therapeutic alliance	Y	Y	Y	Y
Treatment goal consensus	Y	Y	Y	Probably
Collaborative agreement on how to achieve agreed upon goals	Y	Y	Y	Probably
Empathy and validation	Y	Y	Y	Y
Treatment model features				
Well-structured treatment	Y	Y	Y	? Moderately
Active therapist	Y	Y	Y	Modestly active
Regularly scheduled sessions for adult treatments	Y	Y	N/A	Y
Clinician monitoring and quality assurance	Y	Y	Y	Y
Treatment model that one believes in, has clear focus, and is theoretically principled and coherent	Y	Y	Y	Y
Supervision/team	Y	Y	Y	Y
Self-observation—therapist	Y	Y	Y	Y
Skills in managing suicidality, including balanced response	Y	Y	Y	Y
Self-observation—client	Y	Y	Y	Y
Identifying emotions	Y	Y	Y	Y
Analysis of events leading up to and following events	Y	Y	Y	Y
Additional topics not discussed in chapter text				
Treatment manual	Y	Y	Y	Y
Assessment	Y	Y	Y	Y
Diagnosis shared	Y, 'sensitively'	?	Y, with cautious optimism'	Y

(*continued*)

Table 2.1 (*Continued*)

	SCM	GPM	GCC	SP
Sessions regularly scheduled	Y	Y	Flexible	Y
Family involvement	Y	?	Y++	?
Support	Y	Y	Y	Y
Positive transference left alone	?	Y	?	Y
Medication as adjunct	Y	Y	Y	Y
Medication goal explicitly includes avoiding undue side effects	Y	Y	Y	?
Acute hospitalization goal: brief goal directed	Y	Y	Y	?
General psychiatric review built in	Y	Y	Y	?
Clear organizational structures	Y	Y	Y	?
Promote treatment planning	Y	Y	Y	?
Treatment plans	Y	Y	Y	?
Crisis contact availability with therapist during usual hours	Y	Y	Y	?
Crisis service availability coordinated after hours	Y	Y	Y	?
Promote crisis planning	Y	Y	Y	?
Present day focus	Y	Y	Y	?
Problem-solving skills	Y	?	Y	Probably not
Client outcome evaluation clinically built in	Y, via supervision	Y, formally	Y, via team meeting	?
Assertive outreach for nonattenders	Y	?	Y, early in treatment	?
Case management	Y	Y	Y	Probably not
Advocacy where indicated named	Y	?	Y	?
Support seeking housing/finance/vocation where relevant named	Y	?	Y	Probably not

Y, Yes; N/A, not applicable.

contexts, being designed to deliver standardized high-quality treatments considered to be achievable in economically developed countries. This chapter elucidates and clarifies the common features of the treatments and suggests what the active ingredients of change might be.

Zanarini (2009) writes that in treating people with BPD it may be "that any reasonable treatment provided by reasonable people in a reasonable manner may be beneficial." In this chapter, by looking at the features common to four effective evidence-based generalist treatments, we explore what might constitute an effective "reasonable treatment provided by reasonable people in a reasonable manner" that will be superior to the ineffective or harmful historical treatments-as-usual provided in the past.

In the book that arose from the American Psychological Association Division 29 Task Force on Psychotherapy, Horvath and Bedi (2002) state, "a very large part of what is helpful for clients receiving psychotherapy is shared across diverse treatments. It is logical, therefore, that attention should focus on the pantheoretical or generic factors shared by different therapeutic modalities."

This chapter looks at the pantheoretical factors shared by four generalist treatments shown to be effective in treating people with BPD. The effectiveness demonstrated in research of these four treatments, carried out in four separate centers in four countries, took the BPD professional world by surprise, and was the catalyst for writing this book.

The effective generalist treatments for BPD

The four generalist treatments that have been shown to be effective are:

SCM

+ London, UK NHS (affiliated with University College, London).
+ Developed by Anthony Bateman, Peter Fonagy, Rory Bolton, and Eric Karas at the Halliwick Unit, St Ann's Hospital, London.
+ Compliant with 2009 NICE UK government guidelines.
+ Treatment "based on a counseling model closest to a supportive approach with case management, advocacy support" and problem-solving, including crisis plans, medication review, and assertive follow-up if sessions missed.
+ Medication as an adjunct as per 2001 American Psychiatric Association (APA) guidelines and NICE UK government guidelines.
+ Treatment provided by nonspecialist clinicians.
+ Frequency of sessions: regular weekly individual and group sessions.

Bateman and Fonagy (2009b), in a randomized controlled trial, compared a specialist treatment (mentalization-based therapy) with a generalist treatment (SCM). Substantial improvements were documented in both treatments across a range of clinical outcome measures. Mentalization-based therapy achieved steeper and somewhat larger effect sizes after 18 months but SCM was as effective over the initial 6 months and faster at reducing self-harm.

GPM

- Toronto, Canadian public health care system (affiliated with the University of Toronto).
- Developed by Paul Links, Yvonne Bergmans, Jon Novick, and Jeannette LeGris.
- Based on and compliant with the 2001 APA guidelines.
- Treatment: psychodynamically informed psychotherapy, case management and symptom-targeted medication as adjunct using the APA algorithm. Psychodynamic approach drawn from Gunderson (2008), emphasizing early attachment and disturbed attachment as a primary deficit.
- Therapy provided by clinicians with "expertise, aptitude and interest" (McMain et al., 2009) in the treatment of BPD (66% were psychiatrists).
- Frequency of sessions: 1 hour weekly.

McMain et al. (2009), in a randomized controlled trial, compared a specialist treatment (DBT) to a generalist treatment (GPM) in treating clients with BPD over 1 year. The client sample was of significant severity and the DBT and GPM treaters were rated as adherent. The study found GPM and DBT to be equally effective at the end of treatment with significant improvements documented across a range of clinical outcome measures. No differences between treatments were found at 2 year follow-up (McMain et al., 2012).

GCC

- Melbourne, Australian government-funded public mental health service (affiliated with the University of Melbourne).
- Manual developed by Andrew Chanen, Louise McCutcheon, Dominic Germano, and Helen Nistico (Chanen, McCutcheon, Germano, & Nistico, 2000).
- Cognitive-behaviourally informed using a problem-solving paradigm as the core treatment intervention plus high value placed on effective organizational structures.
- Cognitive-behaviourally trained clinical psychologists provided both the therapy and case management, all clients had a psychiatrist on team, and all clients discussed weekly in team meeting.
- Frequency of contact: median contacts/week 1.3; therapy sessions flexible up to a maximum of 24 sessions over 6 months (mean 11 50-minute sessions). In addition, flexible case management sessions (mean 2.9 for every

therapy session) "highlighting that intervention involves more than just formal psychotherapy" (Chanen et al., 2008).

Chanen et al. (2008, 2009), in a randomized controlled trial, compared a specialist treatment (cognitive analytic therapy) with a generalist treatment (GCC) for adolescents with BPD or BPD traits. The study found GCC and cognitive analytic therapy to be generally equally effective with significant improvements documented across a range of clinical outcome measures.

SP

- US metropolitan area that included three eastern US states; private office community practice.
- Developed by Ann Appelbaum and Monica Carsky, drawn partially from previous work by Larry Rockland (Rockland, 1992).
- Strong emphasis on establishing and maintaining a comfortable relaxed therapy relationship with minimal use of interpretation.
- "Provides emotional support-advice on the daily problems facing the patient .... The therapist follows and manages the transference but explicitly does not use interpretations" (Clarkin et al., 2007). The fundamental vehicle of change is seen as the client identifying with the therapist's consistent attitudes towards them of benevolence, interest, kindness, and nonjudgmental acceptance (Appelbaum, 2006).
- Frequency of sessions: weekly supplemented with additional sessions as required.

Clarkin et al. (2007), in a randomized controlled trial, compared three treatments for people with BPD carried out over 1 year. The three treatments comprised two different specialist treatments (transference-focused psychotherapy and DBT) and one generalist treatment (SP). The study found that all three treatments resulted in significant improvements across a range of clinical outcome measures with outcomes across the three treatments being "generally equivalent" (Clarkin et al., 2007). The SP treatment had just one scheduled session/week plus additional sessions if required whereas the two specialist treatments had two scheduled sessions/week. No data on actual resources used and DBT adherence could be found in the study's publication.

International BPD experts

Bateman and Fonagy (2000) name the following features that they believe important in effective treatments for people with BPD: well-structured treatment, a treatment theory that is coherent, clear focus of treatment goals, active clinician, encouragement of a powerful attached therapy relationship, monitoring of treatment and clinician competencies, and integration with other services. More recently Bateman (2012) summarized effective treatments as (a) providing a structure through their manual which supports the therapist and provides recommendations for common clinical problems, (b) being structured so that they encourage increased activity, proactivity, and self-agency for the patients, (c) focusing on emotion processing, particularly on creating robust connections between acts and feeling, (d) increasing cognitive coherence in relation to subjective experience in the early phase of treatments by the inclusion of a model of pathology that is carefully explained to the patient, and (e) encouraging an active therapist stance which invariably includes an explicit intent to validate and demonstrate empathy and generates a strong attachment relationship to create a foundation of alliance.

Gunderson and Links (2008) name the following features that they believe are important in effective treatments for people with BPD: structure, contracting, monitoring clinician competencies and practice, client encouraged to link emotions and actions, BPD-specific clinician training and experience, highly active and involved clinician, clinician qualities of good affect tolerance, empathy, and self-sufficiency, attending to clinician countertransference, and clinician supervision and/or consultation.

Paris (2008) names the following, which he believes are common ingredients of all effective psychological treatments: therapy alliance, empathy, and problem solving. Paris (2010) states the following features that he believes are likely to be particularly important for effective treatment for people with BPD: structure, validation and empathy, and client self-observation.

Zanarini (2008) names three core areas she believes are common to the effective treatment of people with BPD: lessening client pain in part by the judicious use of validation, clarification of bilateral inaccurate communications, and future orientation that values life outside of therapy as a major forum for repair and recovery. The latter view is supported by psychotherapy outcome research meta-analyses showing that factors outside therapy account for approximately the same amount of change as factors inside therapy (Lambert & Barley, 2002).

Weinberg et al (2011) developed a treatment interventions rating scale rating the presence or absence of an intervention in manuals of six separate evidence-based BPD treatments, including five specialist treatments and one generalist treatment (GPM). They named the following features as being present across all treatments: clear treatment framework ("to orient patients to therapy and to elicit responsible attitudes towards maintaining workable treatment relationships"), attention to affect (seeing emotion as being on pathway to problem behavior, accepting and tolerating painful emotion), focus on treatment relationship (including therapist relating as engaged "real" person), active therapist, explorative interventions, and change-oriented interventions.

Commonalities of the effective generalist treatments for BPD

Method

In determining commonalities, we initially included only features that were clearly articulated in the respective manuals, resulting in a narrow range of topics. We decided that this more rigorous approach, resulting in a narrow range of topics, suitable perhaps for an article, would deprive this chapter of clinically useful material. As this book is deliberately and unashamedly practical and clinical, we decided to trade off some possible loss of accuracy in favor of increased clinical utility by including also those features that we felt could reasonably be assumed to exist based on the reading of the manuals. We acknowledge the inherent scientific weaknesses herein.

Three of the four treatments (SCM, GPM, and GCC) were public service team-based treatments with the fourth treatment (SP) being private individual treatment. All treatments were carried out in real-world clinical settings. For ease of reading, we have chosen not to identify each time that a feature of the public service team-based treatments does not apply to the private individual treatment, assuming that readers will be able to discern obvious context differences.

Language

The four treatment manuals understandably sometimes use their own language, so we have either coopted language from one or more of the manuals or have used our own language where we have felt that this best bridged the four treatments.

Literature providing treatment details and manuals

Readers interested in implementing or wanting further descriptive detail about one or more of these treatments are referred to Appelbaum (2006, 2008), Chanen et al. (2009), Kolla et al. (2009), and the APA guidelines (2001). This book includes all the information contained in the original SCM manual used in the research study and more.

Categories

We have conceptually divided common aspects of treatment into the following categories: initial therapeutic stance, therapy relationship, and treatment model features (including supervision/team, clinician monitoring, and skills in managing suicidality).

Initial therapeutic stance

Research shows a sizable contribution of client expectancy of treatment outcome to psychotherapy treatment outcome (Norcross, 2002) replicated in people with BPD (Wenzel, Jeglic, Levy-Mack, Beck, & Brown, 2008). The APA's Division 29 Psychotherapy Task Force comment that clients having a positive expectancy of treatment is thought in meta-analysis research to account for 25% of intratherapy change. In the only study specifically of people with BPD, Wenzel et al. (2008) demonstrated positive client expectancy of treatment outcome predicted treatment outcome. Willing, welcoming, enthusiastic, and hopeful clinicians and organizations will maximize this expectancy dimension of therapeutic change as well as optimizing their own direct effectiveness.

Clinicians who choose to work with people with BPD

Working with people with BPD is recognized as a difficult and challenging area, where optimizing as many facets of treatment as possible will enhance clinical outcomes. For this reason, we believe that it is wise for clinicians to voluntarily choose to work with people with BPD. Having clinicians reluctantly treating people with BPD is a recipe for poor client outcomes and clinician burn-out. We support the legitimacy of private clinicians who do not want to do this work to be explicit with prospective clients about not doing it. Where clinicians are part of an organization, clinicians who choose not to work with people with BPD can make an equally valuable organizational contribution by working in other challenging areas within the organization. It is our experience that where organizations provide clinicians with sufficient time to do the work, there are always clinicians who want to work with people with BPD despite, or perhaps because of, the challenges. Research has shown that generalist BPD treatment training can increase clinician willingness to work with people with BPD (Krawitz, 2004).

Clinicians who are enthusiastic about working with people with BPD

To maximize outcomes, we encourage clients to throw themselves with 100% effort into their recovery. To maximize client outcomes, it makes sense then to also have clinicians who will be enthusiastic, energized, and fully committed to the work. Clinicians who choose to work with people with BPD are likely to be far more enthusiastic about their work than clinicians who are doing the work reluctantly.

Clinicians who are hopeful that people with BPD can recover

Hopefulness in the clinician is thought to be a core ingredient of all effective therapies, with hopelessness in both clinician and patient being shown to increase suicide risk in the patient and being shown to be the most important predictor of suicide in depressed people (Wright et al., 2006). Again, research has shown that training general mental health professionals in the treatment of people with BPD increases clinician optimism in working with people with BPD (Krawitz, 2004), probably by giving an understanding of how to structure treatment and by providing the skills outlined in this book.

Clinicians who are welcoming (and compassionate) of BPD clients

Clinicians who enthusiastically choose to work with people with BPD are likely to be welcoming of clients, believing that people with BPD are deserving of compassionate effective treatment. This is likely to promote feelings in the client that they are being taken seriously and that their distress is significant. Histories of perceived and court-documented neglect, criticism, rejection, and abuse are common in people with BPD and therapy should not be a repeat of these past experiences. It is parsimonious to assume that being welcoming will promote the therapeutic alliance and client outcomes. Research has demonstrated lower self-harm rates in the week following a therapy session where clinicians held nonpejorative conceptualizations of their clients (Shearin & Linehan, 1994). Research has also shown that clinicians' compassionate views of their clients is predictive of positive client outcomes (Henry, Schacht, & Strupp, 1990). Validation and empathy, both effective interventions, are likely to be enhanced when clinicians have a compassionate attitude towards their clients, looking to understand the functions and drivers of their behavior and distress.

Organization willingness

Organizations need to be enthusiastic, hopeful, and welcoming if they are to treat people with BPD; they need to believe that people with BPD are deserving of compassionate effective treatment. Organizational investment in improving treatment for people with BPD is likely to promote clients' feelings that they are being taken seriously and that their distress is being taken seriously. This attitudinal stance will mean that the organization will be more likely to validate the difficulties and challenges of the work clinicians take on by, amongst other things, ensuring that clinicians are given sufficient time, training, support, and supervision to do the work. Where these organizational characteristics are lacking, the person who wants to promote effective treatment in the organization might consider overt use of motivational factors, that is, what are the advantages and disadvantages of the organization being willing to treat people with BPD? Will a willing treatment structure enhance organizational goals of treating high-risk clients, alleviating those with high levels of suffering, reduce suicides, reduce hospitalization rates, reduce complaints, reduce staff burn-out and increase client satisfaction, hospital bed availability and staff morale, and, depending on the context, save money?

Therapy relationship

Meta-analyses of psychotherapy outcome research show that, in general, common factors accounted for twice as much change as specific techniques from different models (Lambert & Barley, 2002). However, some specific treatments, such as exposure treatment of anxiety disorders, accounted for more change than the therapy relationship (Lambert & Barley, 2002). We do not yet have research on what percentage of change is mediated in BPD treatment by the therapy relationship and how much by the techniques of treatment. It seems likely that in treating people with BPD there is a transactional relationship between the model of treatment and the therapy relationship that mediates positive outcomes. In other words, effective models will maximize and enhance the effectiveness of the therapy relationship, which will in turn transactionally maximize and enhance the effectiveness of the model of treatment. Likewise, effective therapy relationships will maximize and enhance the model of treatment, which in turn will transactionally maximize and enhance the effectiveness of the model, and so on, in an upward spiralling transactional manner. The outcome is thus much more than the additive value of the model and the therapy relationship.

Division 29 Task Force on Empirically Supported Therapy Relationships

The APA commissioned the Division 29 Task Force on Empirically Supported Therapy Relationships to look at research of what works in general in therapeutic relationships, culminating in a 450-page publication (Norcross, 2002). The Task Force Steering Committee concluded that the following were "demonstrably effective" features of effective therapy: "therapeutic alliance, cohesion in group therapy, empathy and goal consensus and collaboration." The Task Force concluded that the following were "promising or probably effective": positive regard, congruence/genuineness, feedback, repair of alliance ruptures, self-disclosure, management of countertransference, and quality of relational interpretations. The Task Force's practice recommendations included creating and cultivating a therapeutic relationship that routinely monitored client responses to the treatment and to the therapy relationship, stating, "Such monitoring increases opportunities to repair alliance ruptures, to improve the relationship, to modify technical strategies, and to avoid premature termination" (Steering Committee, 2002).

In the area of BPD, Ann Appelbaum, (Appelbaum, 2006), who developed the SP manual, writes, before the study's later data analysis demonstrated roughly equivalent outcomes across the three treatments, that, "it may come as no surprise to seasoned clinicians and researchers alike, if the harvest of results amounts to what most of us already believe, that the general skill of the clinician and the match between patient and clinician have much more to do with the long-range outcome than the particular technique being applied."

Therapeutic alliance

Bateman et al. (2009a) describe the alliance as having three components: therapy relationship bond, joint understanding of treatment methods, and agreement regarding therapy goals. Horvath and Bedi (2002) include as part of the alliance: mutual liking, respect, and caring, commitment to the goals of therapy, and partnership where both parties are enthusiastic about their respective responsibilities. We view alliance as a clinician activity that can be conscious and purposeful.

Horvath and Bedi (2002), in reviewing for the APA the effect of alliance on psychotherapy outcomes, state that the effect size of the alliance on outcome is about 0.23, "far in excess" of the outcome accounted for by technique. Whilst it seems likely, we do not yet know whether or how much these conclusions can be extrapolated to the specific area of BPD.

It is our belief that positive alliance is maximized when individuals and organizations believe in the right of clients to effective compassionate treatments and are welcoming of seeing such clients. Hopefulness and enthusiasm will arise out of and suffuse these treatment contexts.

Alliance is likely to be promoted by a clinician stance of interest, curiosity, respect, warmth, positive regard, openness, and flexibility. Some of these features could be conceptually linked with liking our clients and the notion of being an active "engaged real" person outlined by Weinberg et al. (2011). Not liking our clients will be normative in our work on occasions and a situation that we can reasonably predict. Whilst these times might be normative, they are likely to be extremely corrosive of the therapy relationship and the therapy alliance, such that early action needs to be taken to prevent premature termination by either party, or a relationship that continues but is not therapeutic. At these times we will endeavor to assess the situation, including self-reflection, and take the matter to supervision and team discussion, often heralded by comments such as "Please help me with increasing my empathy and compassion for my client" or "Please help me assess what needs to be different in the therapy." It is our belief that clinicians' prior commitment to work on situations of "not liking the client" will promote effective outcomes for both client and clinician. Appelbaum (2006) writes, "The therapist must find a way to respect and like the patient and to be genuinely interested: being disliked does not feel safe; and indifference is even more toxic. When therapists are unable to like and care about the patient, the on-going supervision group ... is usually able to help them understand the negative feelings and correct them."

Alliance rupture is fairly normative or nearly universal at some stage, at least in treating people with BPD, and "should be seen as an opportunity to develop the relationship rather than an occasion to end the treatment" (Bateman & Fonagy, 2009a). Whilst as clinicians we proactively aim to prevent alliance ruptures, when they inevitably occur, they might well provide not only the greatest challenge for our clients and ourselves but also the greatest opportunities for learning for both parties. In orienting clients to treatment we predict alliance ruptures and make an overt commitment ourselves to our clients to work hard on repair when this occurs and seek out the same commitment from our clients. In our opinion, this psychoeducation and commitment to work on future relationship difficulties promotes the opportunity aspects of future alliance rupture. Bateman et al. (2009b), in their SCM manual, state that when alliance rupture occurs the clinician will revisit the treatment rationale, seek out and clarify misunderstandings, and refocus on tasks and goals relevant to the client.

Alliance as treatment goal consensus and collaborative agreement on how to achieve these goals

Client and clinician commitment to the goals of therapy and how to go about achieving these goals are included in both Bateman et al.'s (2009a) and Horvath and Bedi's (2002) definitions of alliance. The process of collaboration and shared decision-making is particularly challenging in working with people with BPD. Meta-analysis of general psychotherapy outcome studies supports the value of goal consensus and related collaboration as a factor in achieving positive outcomes (Tryon & Winograd, 2002).

Clinicians', assessing the stage of change that clients are in, will promote goal consensus and collaboration by engaging in behavior congruent with the client's stage of change (Miller & Rollnick, 2002; Prochaska, Norcross, & Diclemente, 1994). Treatment goal consensus and collaboration with clients at the contemplation stage of change is likely to be increased by clinicians and clients focusing on the advantages and disadvantages of change, whereas in the action stage, goal consensus and collaboration will be increased by clinicians and clients focusing on how change may be achieved practically.

Empathy and validation

Validation of a client happens when a clinician communicates to the client that their experience or action is correct (as judged by scientific or community consensus), effective, reasonable or understandable *and the client is in agreement*. The client will have the experience that the clinician "gets it." Three-part empathy includes the clinician knowing the client's experience and communicating this knowing to the client, and the client receiving the communication as making sense. It is not sufficient for us as clinicians to be empathic and to make what we consider empathic, compassionate, and validating responses, but rather that our clients receive these communications as empathic, validating, and compassionate. To maximize validation and empathy, clinicians will have an awareness of their own sometimes conflicted cognitive and emotional experiences (countertransference). Validation and empathy are recognized as important ingredients of all effective therapies, but are likely to be even more critical in the treatment of people with BPD because of the difficulty of providing consistent clinician responses that are experienced by clients as validating and empathic.

Treatment model features

Treatment that is well structured

SCM, GPM, and GCC are all definitely well-structured generalist treatments with SP probably well-structured. All of these treatments are manualized to assist the structuring of the treatment. International BPD experts name a well-structured treatment as amongst the top features that they believe occur in effective treatments for BPD (Bateman & Fonagy, 2000; Gunderson, 2008; Paris, 2008). It seems that many or most people with BPD, at least in the earlier stages of treatment, are unable to effectively take on the task of structuring their own treatment, as their lives and mind states are not sufficiently stable. This means that clinicians need to provide this necessary structure, at least until such time as the client is consistently stable enough to take charge of providing their own structure to therapy. As clients progress in their recovery, they take an increasingly dominant role in determining the nature of their therapy and recovery, as is common in therapy with people with less severe conditions.

Active clinicians as structure and more

SCM, GPM, and GCC all promote an active clinician and SP a modestly active clinician. By consensus of expert opinion, treatment of people with BPD has definitely moved away from the opaque observing and reflecting treatments of the past, which appear anecdotally to have been generally ineffective or worse. We believe an active clinician provides much needed structure. An active clinician promotes a relationship that is more likely to be experienced by clients as genuinely interested rather than indifferent. That is, a person who is interested in alleviating another's suffering is likely to be active.

Research on BPD facial recognition suggests that people with BPD are skilful at accurately assessing emotion from facial expression, except for neutral faces where bias towards interpreting negative emotion occurs (Dyck et al., 2009). This suggests that active clinicians being their authentic selves, rather than a clinician persona, might promote accurate communication and an alliance. A deliberately neutral therapist face might be like throwing petrol onto burning embers.

Regularity of scheduled sessions as structure for adult treatments

Clients in all three of the adult generalist treatments had regular scheduled weekly sessions (SCM, GPM, SP), with additional sessions as required built into the SP manual. The three generalist research studies treating adults with BPD ranged from 12 months' (GPM, SP) to 18 months' (SCM) duration.

The GCC study, in which adolescents with BPD traits or a full BPD diagnosis were treated, was of 6 months' duration and had flexible session times. Many adolescent experts promote duration of treatment that is shorter than experts recommend for treating adults. Reasons for this include the less entrenched nature of the condition in adolescents, eagerness to promote a life after therapy, and a time-frame to which adolescents will realistically commit (6 months represents a large percentage of an adolescent's life).

The time-frames named here for adults are those determined by research needs and do not necessarily represent optimal clinical time-frames. It is our belief that for adults, regularly scheduled sessions are effective because they provide structure whilst allaying client abandonment concerns.

Clinician monitoring and quality assurance

We repeat here the APA Division 29 Task Force on Empirically Supported Therapy Relationships practice recommendations to routinely monitor client responses to the treatment and to the therapy relationship, "Such monitoring increases opportunities to repair alliance ruptures, to improve the relationship, to modify technical strategies, and to avoid premature termination" (Steering Committee, 2002).

In the research studies, three of the generalist treatments (GPM, GCC, SP) formally monitored clinician adherence to the standards set in their respective manuals. The fourth treatment (SCM) monitored adherence via supervision. GPM provided clinicians with regular qualitative weekly feedback on adherence monitoring plus annual empirical quantitative adherence data. GCC clinicians were involved in weekly quality assurance of relevant task completion (assessment, risk assessment, management planning, attendance, engagement). GPM clinicians also received an annual consultation from one of three internationally recognized BPD experts.

Monitoring and quality assurance brings clinician activities into sharp awareness and focus of attention, which arguably promote clinician capabilities and competencies. This is one of Bateman and Fonagy's (2000) named features of effective BPD treatment. It is our experience that enthusiastic clinicians who choose to do this work are keen to attend trainings and be part of supervision and team structures that support and maximize their competencies. Alongside this, our experience is that clinicians are anxious about others monitoring their adherence to standards. Possible ways of addressing this are by having clinicians monitor their own adherence standards (as in GPM) or by creating a culture where the perceived value of adherence monitoring and quality assurance outweighs the perceived disadvantages.

Treatment model that one believes in, has clear focus, and is theoretically principled and coherent

The four generalist treatments all have a clear focus on therapy tasks and goals that are readily understood by clinician and client. As these tasks are different across the four treatments, it is likely that it is the clear focus of a *model* that is principled and internally coherent, onto which one can input information, that is the common mediating factor. Providing clients with a sound coherent rationale will promote the expectancy effect previously described (Wenzel et al., 2008). The manuals of the treatments, whilst obviously different, are likely to have promoted this clear focus on a model.

A theoretically coherent model needs to be clinically practical and include a framework for flexibly dealing with and responding to therapy situations as they arise. This will be particularly critical in situations of crisis, suicidality, therapy relationship rupture, and therapy that is stuck. It is at these times very easy for both parties to become overly anxious, resulting in suboptimal clinician and client behavior that may include clinicians inadvertently reinforcing suicidal behavior. At these challenging times, both parties, but especially clinicians, need to step back and seek the wisdom of their theoretically coherent model to guide responsive, flexible, and skilful action, rather than unskillful automatic reaction.

Supervision/team

All four generalist treatments included a team and/or supervision pathway to support clinicians emotionally and to promote clinician effectiveness. Linehan initially incorporated a team approach into her DBT studies for research reasons, and then, based on her experiences, realized that this was an essential clinical ingredient of the treatment package. GPM developers describe the aims of their supervision group as being to anchor clinicians to the approach, to problem solve around clinical dilemmas, to provide a safe environment to discuss countertransference issues, and to attend to administrative issues (Kolla et al., 2009).

The difficulties of the clinical work require mechanisms to be in place to maintain clinician enthusiasm and to prevent burn-out; collegial supervision and/or a team approach are two such mechanisms. When our clients are not doing well, as clinicians we are vulnerable to challenges to our belief in the work and our professional self-esteem. The roles of colleagues include supporting clinician morale by being removed just enough to be able to see the therapy from a meta or macro position, and not getting lost in any particular micro situation of hopelessness. Colleagues can validate the importance of the work when clinicians despair about the value of what they are doing. Colleagues can validate clinicians when clients are not validating or are invalidating of clinicians. Clinician self-compassion has been associated with positive client outcomes (Henry et al., 1990) and colleagues can support our efforts at self-compassion.

Some of the difficulty of the work is that clients may engage in behaviors that reward clinicians for ineffective behaviors and punish clinicians for effective behaviors. This can result in clinicians inadvertently reinforcing client suicidality. Colleagues can counter this by reinforcing effective clinician behaviors.

Having colleagues supervise us to assess our performance for the organization or being mandated in our team to assess our performance for the organization is likely to restrict sharing, suggesting that somewhere as clinicians we need to have a supervision or team space where we are not subject to organizational performance appraisal.

We suggest that as clinicians we need to create an environment where we take appropriate risks to enhance our development and that of our colleagues. Risks involve sharing a "not knowing" stance that inherently acknowledges that we can probably do better, and that others may know better how to respond to a situation than we do. Errors or perceived errors may be shared in the interests of clinician improvement.

Self-observation—clinician

We use the term "clinician self-observation" to describe some of the areas covered by the psychodynamic term "countertransference" when used in its broadest sense. Clinician self-observation is definitely part of the GPM and SP manuals, and almost certainly part of SCM and GCC treatment models. Given the interpersonal transactional nature of the work and the emotional challenges facing clinicians working with people with BPD, it is likely that clinicians who can skillfully observe their own experience and actions will be well placed to be more effective in their treatment of people with BPD. This reflective clinician self-observation is balanced with all four generalist treatments having active rather than passive clinicians, as previously discussed. Related to clinician self-observation are the outcomes of a randomized controlled trial of clinicians-in-training, which demonstrated that clinician mindfulness practice results in better client outcomes (Grepmair et al., 2007).

Skills in managing suicidality, including balanced response to suicidality
The 10% suicide rate in people with BPD means that clinicians, organizations, and treatment models need to take suicidal thoughts, urges, and actions seriously. Alongside this, clinicians must not become overly anxious in a manner that may reduce their skillfulness to manage suicidality; similarly, organizational responses can inadvertently reinforce client suicidal behaviors, for example by becoming overly risk averse. Clinicians and organizations need to be comfortable enough in working with people with a baseline of chronic suicidality and with the episodic acute suicidality that is frequently superimposed and probably universally superimposes in severe forms of BPD. Clinicians and organizations need to communicate explicitly or implicitly to clients that they do not have to be suicidal to be seen. A structure supporting this allows client contact time with clinicians to occur equally to celebrate successes as to respond to crises.

Self-observation

All four generalist treatments include client self-observation as a core treatment intervention. Self-observation is described in different models using language of mentalizing, observing ego, mindfulness, awareness, and behavioral chain analysis, all of which emphasize different facets of self-observation. Allen et al. (2008) devote an entire book to arguing persuasively that client self-mentalizing is central to all effective therapies. Psychodynamic therapies (observing ego), CBT (behavioral chain analysis), and mindfulness- and acceptance-based therapies all also argue persuasively of the central role of client self-observation in effective therapies.

Self-observation deficits using mindfulness measures have been shown to predict BPD features and associated other psychopathology in clinical and nonclinical populations (Wupperman, Neumann, & Axelrod, 2008, 2009). The amount of client self-observation practice using mindfulness practice in a mindfulness-based stress reduction (MBSR) treatment study demonstrated that increased client mindfulness practice resulted in improved outcomes (Carmody & Baer, 2008).

Identifying emotions

Intense emotions leading to counterproductive action are central to the problems of BPD so it makes sense that all the effective generalist treatments encourage client identification of emotions. Emotions are recognized as occurring on the pathway to problem behaviors. Early awareness of emotions promotes skilful client action because emotions can be responded to when they are at a lower level of intensity, making them more manageable. Awareness and labeling of emotions, accepting painful emotion, and tolerating distress decrease automatic client action responses and encourage conscious choices, resulting in increasingly effective behavior.

Analysis of events leading up to and following events, especially sentinel events

All the effective generalist treatments support clinicians and clients collaboratively exploring the internal (thoughts, emotions, body sensations) and external events leading up to and following events, especially sentinel events. This may be via a formal behavioral chain analysis in the cognitive-behaviorally informed generalist treatments or via an open curious wondering of "what happened" in the psychodynamically informed generalist treatments.

How does this relate to effective specialist evidence-based treatments?

It is our belief that the common factors outlined in this chapter are part of all the effective evidence-based specialist treatments for BPD. Do the data that generalist treatments can be effective mean that we should abandon specialist treatments? Our answer is a categorical no! We believe that there will always be important places for both generalist and specialist treatments, and that research data is currently too embryonic to be definitive about what these respective roles will be. It might be that most people with BPD can be successfully treated with a generalist treatment, with a subgroup needing specialist treatment. This applies to treatments for most health conditions. If this is the case, research which identifies who belongs to this subgroup would clearly be beneficial.

Understanding the catalysts of change, clarifying the relative importance of the relationship and techniques in achieving good outcomes, and identifying moderators of outcome would be a major step forward in improving outcomes for people with BPD. Bateman and Fonagy (in press) found that comorbid personality disorder, specifically borderline with Cluster C avoidant personality disorder, reduced the likelihood of a good outcome in mentalization-based therapy but the negative effect was less than for patients treated with structured clinical management. Neacsiu and colleagues (2010) examined the role of DBT skills in improving treatment clinical outcomes. Unsurprisingly, participants treated with DBT reported using three times more behavioral skills by the end of treatment compared to those assigned to a control treatment. However, use of DBT skills mediated the decrease in suicide attempts and depression, and the increase in control of anger, and partially mediated the decrease in nonsuicidal self-injury over time, suggesting that skills acquisition and practice may be an important mechanism of change in DBT. This creates an illusion of a unitary explanation of change across treatments that needs to be avoided if we are to explain how the patients treated with GPM, used in the study comparing DBT with GPM, changed equally and maintained their improvement during follow-up (McMain et al., 2012). It is parsimonious to assume that different treatments will have both common mechanisms of change and also different mechanisms of change.

We do hope that with further research we will be able to achieve better and better outcomes as both generalist and specialist treatments become increasingly more effective. We hope that some of this will occur by cross-fertilization of information between effective treatments. Dismantling studies also will illuminate the way forward, guiding us as a profession as to what needs to be added and what can be left out because it is surplus to effective treatment. We envisage a hopeful future, where at the outset of treatment we will be better able to promote positive outcomes by matching such factors as severity and stage of change with client, clinician, organization, and model characteristics.

Chapter 3

Structured clinical management: general treatment strategies

Summary

Organization of treatment is important. It needs to be well-structured, coordinated, integrated with other services available to the patient, and understandable and predictable to the person with BPD.

Strategic processes include:

+ careful assessment
+ giving the diagnosis
+ information about BPD
+ crisis planning
+ risk assessment and risk management
+ development of a hierarchy of therapeutic areas
+ agreement of clinician and patient responsibilities
+ development of motivation and establishment of therapeutic alliance
+ stabilization of drug misuse and alcohol abuse
+ development and agreement of comprehensive formulation
+ involvement of families, relatives, partners, and others.

In Chapter 2 we discussed the similarities between the evidence-based general psychiatric treatments for BPD that have been used in research trials and specialist approaches. All four treatments, despite being independently developed, show considerable overlap structurally and technically. They are well-organized and carefully planned treatments with an emphasis on methodical, predictable, and reliable delivery of strategies to the patient. Their focus, notwithstanding their more specific therapeutic interventions, on structure and service organization, that is, on how treatment is implemented, indicates the importance placed by experts on general implementation strategies for the successful treatment of people with BPD. Expert consensus suggests that if patients are to benefit from treatment, their experience of the service may be of near equal importance to the specialist techniques used (NICE, 2009). In other words an expertly delivered specialist program will be of limited effectiveness if the service organization and context in which it is offered is chaotic, incoherent, and inconsistent. This is good news for general mental health professionals who have it within their professional competence to structure treatment coherently.

In this chapter and Chapters 4–6 we discuss structured clinical management (SCM), which was used in a research trial as the comparator general psychiatric treatment against which mentalization based therapy was tested (Bateman & Fonagy, 2009b). SCM was developed using expert consensus. Principles considered by experts to represent best general psychiatric treatment for people with BPD were followed. In addition, all interventions had to be within the competence of generalist mental health clinicians or require only limited additional training. Patients in the trial responded well, showing marked improvements in most outcome domains (Bateman & Fonagy, 2009b).

Integrating general treatment strategies into a coherent whole is the first aspect of SCM for patients with BPD. Only once this structural process is robust will the second component of SCM, the clinician working with specifically tailored interventions, have a chance of success.

Structure

Structure describes the way in which a program is put together, how it is implemented on a daily basis, how it is organized over the longer term, how predictable it is, and how clear its boundaries are in terms of roles and responsibilities. Inconsistency, lack of co-ordination, incoherence of response, unreliability, and arbitrariness are all antithetical to structure (Bateman & Fonagy, 2004). Clinicians are used to structuring treatment in their role as a mental health professional. They should continue to do this whilst being aware that patients with BPD are more sensitive and reactive to uncertainty and lack of reliability than other groups of patients. The following list is an outline of some of the most important components of structure:

- Information given to the patient must be clear and unambiguous. Most important is that treatment plans are written down and given to the patient. Written information will include:
  - information about the treatment program and contact numbers
  - dates and times of appointments

- details about access to services, e.g. crisis team and crisis house
- contacts of housing and social support services
- contacts of self-referral agencies.

◆ Good collaboration between clinician, the psychiatrist, and other mental health professionals about the treatment plan is necessary. Ensure a structured and organized approach by arranging a care program meeting at the beginning of treatment.

◆ Regular communication with other mental health professionals involved in the patient's care is necessary, for example if the clinician is working with the patient on reducing their prescribed medication and managing emotional fluctuations psychologically, the psychiatrist should be aware of this.

◆ Avoid changes of staff wherever possible. This is of particular relevance in the treatment of BPD in which change of mental health workers is experienced as a re-enactment of earlier loss and abandonment, and can lead to despair and subsequent drop-out.

◆ As soon as any other professional becomes involved in the care of the patient, their role and how they link with the core treatment team needs to be discussed. This applies, for example, when the patient is admitted to medical or psychiatric hospital, the criminal justice system is involved, or housing support is necessary.

◆ Gradually develop a focus for treatment, for example self harm, relationships or lack of motivation. This focus may change over time but should be adequately defined to form the focus for individual sessions and the problem-solving group sessions.

We will now discuss general treatment strategies in more detail.

Pathway to assessment

Many people who have BPD are unaware that they have it. There is limited information freely available, although this has increased dramatically in the last few years with an explosion in the amount of information available on the internet. We make some suggestions about relevant websites in Chapter 7. Most mental health services do not promote public information about psychiatric disorders and government organizations rarely have policies to disseminate information about BPD. There are some notable exceptions to this and the National Alliance on Mental Illness (NAMI) in the USA has a BPD awareness month each year.

The paucity of knowledge about BPD and the stigma associated with mental illness results in people with BPD presenting to services with associated problems. Chronic depression or high anxiety are common (Zanarini, et al., 1998; Zanarini, Frankenburg, Hennen, Reich, et al., 2004). This can be confusing to mental health professionals, who tend not to see the elephant in the room but are distracted by the presenting symptoms. They fail to make the diagnosis of BPD, which results in the patient not receiving appropriate treatment. It is therefore important that all clinicians are vigilant about the diagnosis and are able to undertake a basic assessment reliably. Clinicians do not have to be experts but they need a working knowledge of BPD to ensure that they can make a presumptive diagnosis when appropriate and conversely rule out the disorder when it is not present. This is particularly important when assessing patients who have made a suicide attempt or self-harmed. There is an unfortunate tendency to equate self-harm with BPD, yet around 30–40% of patients with BPD do not self harm (Skodol et al., 2002).

Process of assessment and giving the diagnosis

We have already discussed the criteria required to make a formal diagnosis, considered some alternative ways of thinking about the criteria, and examined the advantages and disadvantages of giving a diagnosis to a patient, coming down on the side of talking to patients about it (see Chapter 1). Certainly specialist treatments recommend clinicians spend considerable time talking to patients about their diagnosis and there is no reason why a well-trained mental health professional cannot do this as part of a generalist treatment. Here we discuss giving the diagnosis to the patient. To do so it is important first to know about personality disorder itself. Second it is necessary to be able to give the diagnosis in a way that engenders hope of change and is relevant to the individual, e.g. by using examples from the patient's life.

Information for the clinician: what is personality disorder?

A person has a personality disorder when the features of his personality show a certain number of maladaptive personality traits, which are generally defined as typical ways of thinking, feeling, managing impulses, and relating to other people. The traits need to have been characteristic of the person since at least late adolescence or early adulthood and have been relatively consistent over time (American Psychiatric Association, 1994). Clinically, as we outlined in Chapter 1, patients with borderline personality subjectively feel that they do not know who they are and that they can change suddenly. Clinicians must recognize that impairment in identity and sense of self, emotion dysregulation, and a low capacity for effective interpersonal functioning are the core of the problem. Of course this begs questions about what a sense of self is, what identity consists of, what emotion dysregulation is, and how we determine effective interpersonal functioning. For example, someone with antisocial personality disorder may have a stable sense of self and a clear identity and be effective in their current social and interpersonal context. However, the same is unlikely to be true for someone with BPD.

Identity

Identity is the experience of oneself as unique and as having a clear distinction between oneself and others. Other individuals are recognized as having different experiences and ideas from our own; one's own experience is not generalized to all others. The individual with a clear identity has a linear sense of time and gives a personal history with a coherent narrative, shows a stability and accuracy of self-appraisal and self-esteem, and describes a capacity for a range of regulated emotional experience. Problems in these areas are characteristic of BPD.

The individual with BPD is uncertain about who she is and often feels she has to be the person someone else wants her to be. She may be chameleon like, fitting in to her surroundings, which further undermines a senses of who she is. Consequently self-direction is poor and ability to be self-reflective is limited. Whilst all this sounds pejorative it need not be so. People with BPD recognize that they lose control of a sense of who they are and are aware that they can be easily influenced by others. They recognize that they can engage in destructive relationships and they often see such features of their life as a problem. The mental health professional who is able to empathize with a person's subjective experience of uncertainty about who she is will be able to talk to her about the problem sympathetically.

Instability in sense of self makes it problematic for people with BPD to understand and appreciate others' experiences and motivations or to accept their differing perspectives. It is inevitable that this interferes with intimacy, especially in terms of the duration of a relationship. Individuals with BPD show rapidly escalating, impassioned, and heartfelt involvement with others until, for example, a perceived slight occurs, at which point they feel abandoned and betrayed equally powerfully, compelling them to end the relationship.

Impulsivity

Impulsivity is one of the defining criteria of BPD and is thought by some to be most characteristic of the condition (Koenigsberg et al., 2002; Henry et al., 2001; Sanislow et al., 2002). However, the term "impulsivity" is used in many different ways by clinicians. Some use it to describe sensation seeking, suggesting that patients with BPD need high levels of stimulation, others refer to risk taking, whilst others consider lack of planning to be the core element. Finally, an inability to delay gratification, insensitivity to consequences of action, and an alteration in the perception of time (Coffey et al., 2011; McCloskey et al., in press) may also be features of impulsivity. It has been pointed out (Coffey et al., 2011) that not only do BPD and substance abuse frequently co-occur, impulsivity is a core feature of both disorders and may be a causal link in the co-occurrence. In part this is why SCM places some emphasis on links with drug and alcohol services (see section on comorbidity in Chapter 6). The clinician needs to discuss each of these aspects of impulsivity with the patient. We suggest that clinicians ask specific questions about each area:

- Do you tend to seek out pursuits that give a heightened sensory experience and involve risk?
- Do you plan what you do and think about the different outcomes?

Consumer comment

I don't care about what happens. I can take a decision based on how I feel at that moment. When my colleague was critical of me I thought that I had had enough so I went back to my room, booked a flight to Greece on the internet, sent an e-mail resigning, and left.

Emotion dysregulation

Emotion dysregulation (Gratz, 2007) refers to unskillful actions that are consequent on strong and often overwhelming emotion and includes much of what is described above on impulsivity.

Interpersonal

In Chapter 1, following the descriptive criteria for BPD, we outlined the instability, intensity, and sensitivity of relationships (Gunderson & Lyons-Ruth, 2008), which are characterized by extremes of idealization and devaluation in BPD. As a clinician engaged in implementing SCM it is necessary to identify a number of former and current relationships of the patient. Explore their quality and pinpoint any patterns. Patterns are important because they indicate the possible trajectory of treatment. Unstable relationships characterized by overcloseness followed by sudden detachment, for example, do not augur well for a smooth treatment course. Furthermore, clarifying detail of what happens in the relationships of the patient will reveal potential sensitivities within interpersonal situations, providing information to be used in any crisis plan. Crises in patients with BPD often start within an interpersonal interaction due to the hypersensitivity of their attachment processes.

Consumer comment

I don't do relationships any more. They are bad for me and they always go wrong. I can't keep falling in love with people so I am trying to keep away from all those parties I used to go to. When someone shows that they fancy me I think that I am a star and I am on the top of the world but I know now that that is a dangerous feeling so I avoid people.

Interpersonal sensitivity

The hypervigilance of people with BPD is well-documented and is not surprising given the developmental experiences of most patients. It is important not to suggest to patients that their experience of reality is unreal, as very often they will accurately perceive the negative attitude of others. Their problem is linked more to the strength of their reaction when they feel misunderstood or devalued or disliked than it is to inaccurate perception, and they feel misunderstood more frequently than most. In essence patients have two reactions: they become overwhelmed with feeling or they become detached. Neither helps them process the problem and both are disproportionate to the context. Ask the patient if they ever experience a sudden feeling of distrust when with others. Let them know that many people can be thin-skinned and ask if they think they can be sensitive or oversensitive to what others are saying or thinking. These and other questions to ask the patient when considering the different problem areas in BPD are summarized as follows:

Questions to ask a patient when exploring areas of personality function:

+ What makes you you?
+ Does your sense of who you are change?
+ Do you know who and what you like and dislike?
+ Do you tend to become what others want you to be?
+ Are you easily influenced by others?
+ Can you tell what other people are thinking?
+ Do you seek out sensation and risky pursuits?
+ Are you a careful planner?
+ Do you think about the consequences of your decisions before you make a final decision?

- Does the intensity of your emotions lead to actions that you later regret?
- How would you describe the quality of your relationships?
- Are you always on the alert when with other people?
- Are you concerned with what others think about you?
- Can you be oversensitive?

Giving the diagnosis

But how does the clinician give the diagnosis in a way that is beneficial and helpful? This is less of a problem with patients who show BPD that is noncomorbid with other personality disorders, although even then it may be difficult. But it becomes more difficult if the patient is comorbid for borderline, narcissistic, paranoid, and antisocial personality disorder and also has an Axis I disorder. The clinician cannot hide behind the failings of nosology, pass responsibility, and blame inadequate diagnostic systems, or simply say that we do not believe in diagnosis. Even if the clinician does not believe in categorical diagnostic systems, someone else in the mental health service, perhaps the emergency service, might have said that "they have a personality disorder which is untreatable." Uncertainty and doubt about the value of diagnosis may be appropriate but avoidance and lack of clarity is likely to induce distrust in the patient about the competence of the clinician and make the development of a therapeutic alliance more difficult. So we recommend giving the diagnosis as one of the first general therapeutic strategies.

Let us assume that you are taking a categorical approach to personality and have concluded that the patient has BPD. In our experience the best approach is to be direct and explanatory, bearing in mind that you want to stimulate the patient's capacity to reflect on herself and on your perspective about her. There are many ways to go about this and we do not presume to have the correct answer. If clinicians have better ways of explaining the diagnosis, they should keep to what they do. However, the primary purpose of giving the diagnosis is to stimulate the patient to consider all aspects of herself and for her to reflect on your thoughts about her whilst you demonstrate your capacity to consider her problems.

During the assessment process many of the features of BPD will have become apparent. The task of the assessor is to talk to the patient about the diagnosis in a way that makes it personal to them and generates sustained coherence of their disparate symptoms and subjective experiences. It is often best to outline the four main problem areas of BPD (see Chapter 1) to the patient, giving an example from their life to illustrate what is meant by difficulties in interpersonal relationships, emotional regulation, impulse control, and sensitivity to others. A number of questions (see the list above under interpersonal sensitivity) to the patient about each area can help, asking them to give further examples—Are there other aspects of your relationships which you think cause trouble? How do you manage your emotions? Do you take sudden decisions without considering the consequences? Is the main problem for you when you are with others or when you are on your own? Can you become oversensitive to other people? Do you worry about their motives?

Before giving the diagnosis tell the patient that it has been helpful to get a full picture of them—"I think that I have a good idea how I might describe you now as a person. Can I put it to you so that you can comment?" Then summarize your perspective and ask them to correct you as you progress. Ask the patient for her view of herself. How does she describe herself as a person? When possible, challenge persistent externalization of problems, for example when the patient blames everyone else for her problems. Make sure you say that having a personality disorder does not mean that the entire personality is affected. People have many good and positive personality traits even when they have characteristics that dominate the way they are with other people. Individuals can be extremely talented and have a personality disorder. For example, Edvard Munch clearly suffered from a personality disorder, forming fractious personal relationships with other people. But he was an extremely skilful and innovative painter.

When giving the diagnosis it is necessary frequently to check out the patient's understanding of what you are saying. If you assume too much you will induce defensiveness or if too little you will be challenged as patronizing. The point is not to "tell" the patient what you know and to demonstrate the extent of your knowledge but to stimulate reflection about the problem areas. You are not trying to persuade the patient of your viewpoint.

Once the process of discussing the diagnosis is complete, clinicians need to address immediate issues and the generic strategy that gives the most "bang for the buck" is good crisis planning. This is an area neglected in general mental health settings despite the current emphasis on making risk assessments on all patients.

Consumer comment

I had never heard of the diagnosis borderline personality disorder. I didn't like the idea that I was personality disordered although everyone had always said I was a difficult person. I went home and looked it up on the internet. Wow! It described all the things that were really me. I went straight into a chat room and found all these people who had the same experiences as me. At last I wasn't on my own!

Crisis planning

All patients with BPD will experience crises during treatment. In fact for many mental health professionals their experience of patients with BPD primarily comes from seeing them during a crisis. Recurrent crises are exhausting for everyone involved and lead to burn-out in both patients and staff, so time spent on developing a crisis plan is time well spent.

Developing a crisis plan with a patient is possibly one of the most effective general therapeutic strategies for people with BPD (Borschmann, Henderson, Hogg, Phillips, & Moran, 2012). Hence it is included in our top ten resource-efficient treatment strategies in Chapter 8. Many patients will have tried to access services as an emergency on numerous occasions only to find that their needs have not been met or, worse still, have been exacerbated by the reactions of mental health professionals.

The process of addressing how a patient will interact with services in the future is soothing and reassuring to a patient when done well. The resulting formulation will later form an important aspect of general psychiatric treatment, giving the clinician a specific treatment strategy when crises occur— *"Revisit the crisis plan when a crisis has occurred."*

Here we will discuss some of the practical aspects of developing a plan (Moran et al., 2010). Remember, it is not adequate solely to tell patients that they can attend the emergency assessment centre or the emergency room even if this does become part of an agreed plan. From their perspective it will be insulting. They will have tried it many times. It is also inappropriate to "give" the patient a plan; it is more fitting to stimulate reflection on how the patient will identify that a crisis is emerging, what action they can take to divert the crisis, what others can do that is helpful, and how services can respond. Once the components of the crisis plan are agreed they are written down, given to the patient and placed in their medical records, and whenever possible given to the local emergency centre.

What signals does the patient have that a crisis is emerging?

Ask the patient to describe at least three examples of crises that have led to self-destructive behavior and/or contact with services. Taking each in turn, spend time attempting to work out early warning signs:

- Was there a particular feeling?
- Was there a behavioral change?
- Were thought patterns different?

Even if a patient cannot answer these questions, the task of attending to what was happening is in itself therapeutic. Empathize with any patient who does not know what happens and finds that her feelings can go from zero to a hundred in milliseconds—*"It just happens and there is nothing that I can do."* Even if this is the case, the clinician needs to work with the patient to find some early warning signs as this aspect of the crisis plan is one of the basic strategies for implementing SCM.

In SCM patients are asked to rate their crises on an escalator with 0 at the bottom of the escalator = control, 1 and 2 = defined by patient and clinician, and 3 at the top of the escalator = crisis point or out of control. The clinician uses clarification techniques, frequently coaxing the patient to rewind their mental processes to points prior to their loss of control, thereby helping them to identify triggers and the effect they have on their internal states. In other words the patient is asked to work methodically on "what makes me vulnerable?"

What can the patient do and not do?

The patient identifies when they could have re-established self-control and what could prevent them from moving on to the next stage towards a crisis. How do you stop the escalator? How do you get off? Strategies that have been helpful in managing emotional crises in the past are identified, for example leaving a provocative situation, telephoning someone if trapped in a feeling of loneliness, or distracting the mind by engaging in an action task such as cooking. The clinician also tries to stimulate the patient to reflect on how others might observe each stage (signals for others), and what others could or should not do that might be helpful. Significant others are invited to sessions to work out this part of the crisis plan jointly.

What can other people do and not do?

How do others know that a crisis is emerging? What might they do to help? Taking the three examples that the patient has provided, the clinician asks her to consider what practical and emotional responses of others would have been helpful and identify those that are unhelpful. Someone else being aware of what not to do might have more traction in a crisis than attempting actively to do something useful. For example, partners may be advised to avoid confrontation, side-step disagreement, and to minimize defensiveness when the patient with BPD is emotional and anxious. This is not the same as simply asking others to accept unwarranted personal attacks. Partners need to choose the time for discussion and an emerging crisis in people with BPD is not one of them. After the patient has carefully defined what her partner or others can do when she feels vulnerable and in danger of reaching the top of the escalator, discuss how she passes on this information to them.

What can services do and not do?

In general terms it is important to minimize the usefulness and effectiveness of services in a crisis. Certainly medical emergency health services are not well organized to manage patients with BPD and personnel are poorly trained to understand the severity of the condition. Sadly the same can be said for many mental health emergency services and the patient is well-advised to keep away from poor-quality mental health emergency services if at all possible. Again, the crisis plan may not so much be about what can the services do but what should they try not to do. For example, crisis presentation is a time when clinicians commonly change medication when it is, in fact, the least sensible time to start altering a prescription. A statement in the crisis plan such as "even if I demand it, please be careful about changing my medication in a crisis. I can consider this later when I am calmer" will help professionals act responsibly rather than out of their own ill-considered panic and need to do something.

The crisis plan is a work in progress and each time certain aspects become clearer they are added to the plan. The clinician is required to revisit the crisis plan whenever a crisis occurs. When agreed actions or psychological techniques fail to stop the escalator they are re-evaluated. In this way the clinician continuously maintains the patient's own responsibility for dealing with painful and possibly overwhelming emotions whilst at the same time strengthening their ability to do so; all along with clinician support.

Having identified possible self-help interventions, the feasibility of implementation over 24 hours, 7 days a week needs to be considered. Many crises will occur in the evenings, at night, or at weekends, when only emergency services are available.

In addition to patient-specific plans, the clinician outlines the emergency system that is available to the patient, emphasizing that emergency teams will have access to the crisis plan whenever possible. Emergency staff will attempt to help the patient manage an acute situation. From there it becomes the responsibility of the patient as much as the emergency staff to contact the treatment team on the next working day. The patient and the case manager may then decide to organize an emergency appointment (lasting no more than 20 minutes wherever possible in order not to reinforce crises inadvertently) to focus entirely on the crisis and on how to stabilize the situation if it recurs. The primary aim is to reinstate psychological and behavioral safety for the patient and others.

Consumer comment

I wrote loads of complaint letters to the hospital about how I was treated. I phoned up the crisis team when I was in crisis. What are they called a crisis team for? They don't do anything in a crisis. I think they hoped I would kill myself as that would get me out of their way. On one occasion they put the phone down on me. I didn't like talking about how I was going to manage myself in a crisis when I had to do this as part of my treatment plan. I thought my psychiatrist should sort out the crisis team so that they did what they were supposed to do. But in the end it was a good idea to see what sort of things I could do myself even though I did it mainly because contacting the crisis team worked me up more. But my shrink also put down what he would do and we agreed stuff between us so it was not all me having to do stuff.

Risk assessment, risk management and legal concerns

Comprehensive risk assessments should be made using the current risk assessment protocol of the hospital. These commonly include information about past and present risks, indicators of increased risk, and factors that decrease risk. The clinician needs to take a detailed history of previous suicide attempts and/or acts of self-harm and other areas of risk. Information from the risk assessment will, of course, inform the crisis plan.

A clinician is likely to feel responsible for a patient who is at high risk to herself, including feeling accountable for keeping her alive (see section on feelings in the clinician in Chapter 6). An active response from a clinician to high suicide risk may be the necessary response for a patient to feel that her risk is taken seriously. All this places the clinician in an invidious position when discussing how to manage the risk of a patient with BPD. What will the clinician do and what will the clinician not do?

Acute and chronic risk

Many patients with BPD are suicidal over long periods of time, with the intensity of their suicidal feeling and thoughts fluctuating on a daily basis. Superimposed on this are times of immediate and high risk, often as a response to a current stressor, when suicidal feelings dominate rather than being in the background (Paris, 2003). The long-term ongoing risk has to be considered throughout treatment and becomes something that is monitored by both patient and clinician, and taken as part of the disorder. Chronic suicidal thoughts become something that the patient "lives with" and the clinician does not take active responsibility for addressing them but considers them in relation to the patient's overall problems, that is, as part of their way of life and the way in which they manage feelings and their experience of the world. Suicide is seen by patients as a solution in the background as an answer to any problem that the patient feels she cannot manage. The clinician works with the patient to find safer and more constructive ways of managing distress. In an acute suicidal crisis the clinician is more active, considering admission to a crisis unit or inpatient facility (see Chapter 6), vigorously supporting the patient on the telephone if necessary, and working specifically on the crisis plan.

Legal aspects

The desire to be responsive to UK clinicians involved in the considerable discussions following a recent controversial court decision resulted in one of us (AB), who is UK based, summarizing the current legal precedents in the UK for clinicians treating suicidal patients with BPD. The discussion is based on an excellent article by David and colleagues (2010).

Most patients will not engage the clinician in a challenging discussion about whether they have the right to take their own life. But some patients will do so and may even defy the clinician's best advice at the point at which they have taken an overdose of tablets and are in danger of death. Whilst this may be rare, it is necessary for the clinician to have some guidance on his responsibility and to have a working knowledge of legal aspects of risk. So I cover this topic here from a UK perspective although the principles and clinical concerns may be relevant in other regions and countries.

UK legal jurisdiction has separated capacity/incapacity legislation on the one hand from mental health legislation on the other. Clinicians need to have a working knowledge of both. In UK law a person lacks capacity in relation to a matter if at the time they are unable to decide for themselves in relation to the matter because of an impairment of, or disturbance in the functioning of, the mind or brain. "Unable" is defined as being unable to understand and retain information relevant to the decision, to use or weight that information in coming to a decision, and to communicate a decision. Importantly, there is a legal assumption of capacity until proven otherwise. Judging someone's decision from a clinical viewpoint as imprudent or reckless, for example, is not adequate to determine incapacity, although a refusal to discuss the reasons for a decision may suggest further investigation of capacity is merited, especially when the likely outcome of the decision is death.

A patient with BPD who takes a life-threatening overdose and then alerts the clinician to the act merits further investigation simply because they have involved another person in the problem. Taking the capacity aspect of the patient first, it is likely that a person with BPD or other severe personality disorder will have capacity unless a comorbid disorder is complicating the picture. Patients with BPD are able to retain information and understand it to the extent that they can consider it to come to a decision. So the essential question falls as to whether or not their BPD, an illness characterized by emotional turmoil, rapid mood changes, and distortions in thinking, might interfere with use of information and even impede balanced decision-making. It is difficult for the clinician to decide this alone and discussion with colleagues is mandatory. In essence the clinician needs at this point to consider not just capacity but the second legal aspect of the problem—does the current severity of the illness suggest detention in hospital is warranted and if so will the use of the Mental Health Act permit necessary life-saving intervention depending on the meaning attributed to treatment in this situation? Courts have allowed the use of nasogastric tubes to give life-saving treatment to patients with anorexia nervosa using the Mental Health Act so it is within the bounds of possibility that inflicting life-saving treatment on a patient with BPD is permissible if the person has a mental disorder warranting detention and treatment under the Mental Health Act for her health and safety.

Given the separation of capacity and mental illness the clinician is faced with a serious dilemma in patients with BPD who may present following a life-threatening act of self-harm but who show capacity and whose acute symptoms of BPD may not be apparent. The emotional balancing properties of self-harm are well known, so a person initially managing an emotional crisis precipitated by an interpersonal conflict may have quickly changed into someone who appears calm, tranquil, and thoughtful. The British courts have considered this situation. In a recent case the court denied clinicians the right to give life-saving treatment to a patient with BPD following her ingestion of antifreeze. She subsequently died. She was considered to have capacity and not to have a mental illness warranting detention.

Despite this judgment I recommend that clinicians act extremely carefully. It is my view that medical treatment should have been given in the acute situation. Readers are advised to investigate legal precedent in their own countries and this report is only a summary of a recent case in the UK. It is included here because it has become a focus for discussion. The decision of the court might have been different if the clinicians had taken into account the individual's history, which is highly relevant when assessing personality disorder. Changes to decisions are characteristic of BPD, acute wishes to die fluctuate as they had in this patient in the past, intentions are responsive to the actions of others, and treatment for the disorder is not hopeless. The clinician is therefore best advised to act safely and do whatever he can to save the patient who attends an appointment stating she has taken a serious overdose and does not want to go to hospital. Talking the patient through this decision, taking care not to be coercive in response to one's own desperation, might be the best therapeutic intervention for the patient in this context. Then call a senior colleague, inform the nearest relatives, and facilitate the patient's transfer to hospital.

Hierarchy of therapeutic areas

Helping a patient break down overwhelming life problems into smaller parts is itself a therapeutic process. Many patients will have aims that are generalized, overambitious, and unachievable in a short time—"I want to get my life back and to feel I know who I am." A patient who says that she wants to have better relationships is making an understandable wish and yet needs to develop a pathway of incremental steps to achieve her goal. What makes a better relationship needs definition; what would have to change to increase the likelihood of positive outcomes in relationships warrants scrutiny.

Similarly, exploration should be given to the other problem areas relevant to people with BPD. We suggest breaking down the therapeutic areas into the four areas of interpersonal relationships, emotional dysregulation, impulsivity, and interpersonal sensitivity. These in turn are subdivided according to the difficulties that the patient has discussed and a hierarchy of areas and subtargets made. These will later form part of the problem-solving aspects of SCM.

The clinician focuses on:

- interpersonal:
  - engagement in therapy by developing a therapeutic alliance despite the alliance being challenged by the interpersonal problems of the patient
- impulsivity:
  - reduction of self-damaging, threatening, or suicidal behavior
  - rash decision-making
- emotional dysregulation:
  - emotional storms
  - crisis demand
- cognitive distortions:
  - interpersonal sensitivity, especially to health service personnel.

Finally, it is important not to miss the severe social consequences that can result from problems associated with these four areas of difficulty. Enquire about accommodation and financial problems, referring the patient to appropriate social support when necessary.

Defining clinician and patient responsibilities

Clarity about clinician and patient responsibilities is essential at the beginning of treatment. The clinician needs to be authentic about what is and what is not possible, taking into account normal professional responsibilities. The patient must be involved in the discussion about the proposed treatment plan so that they can consider different aspects of treatment and agree to the program. Friends, partners, and relatives often know a great deal about the patient's life, interests, and abilities as well as having personal experience of the patient's mental health problems and should be involved in the development of the treatment plan whenever possible. Unless there are over-riding reasons against, the clinician generally accepts to:

- formulate action plans with the patient which are designed to meet problems
- agree timing of subsequent review arrangements
- provide specific information about treatment and its rationale
- engage the patient in the agreed treatment program
- fulfill clinician aspects of an agreed crisis plan
- provide the treatment sessions professionally
- ensure the patient has full information about any medication
- complete and maintain a full risk assessment and treatment plan, which includes the crisis plan
- integrate different components of the patient's involvement with services
- involve patients, carers (family, friends or care staff from residential homes), an independent advocate (if requested), mental health professionals, and others, e.g. police
- document patients' and carers' views on their involvement with the treatment program
- engage other mental health services, housing, and social care when appropriate
- facilitate admission to hospital if necessary.

For their part the patient also agrees to take some responsibilities, which commonly include:

- attending treatment sessions on time
- being open and honest in treatment
- engaging in addressing the agreed target areas
- attempting to stay alive and avoiding acts of self-harm
- fulfilling patient aspects of the crisis plan and revisiting it with the clinician when necessary.

There are a number of ways to ensure workable agreements are developed with the patient. First, the plan has to be meaningful to the patient. Second, it has to be developed collaboratively. Third, it has to address the most painful symptoms and to engender hope that there is a pathway to resolution. This is a process of remoralization. SCM is not coercive but facilitates identification of which of the patient's problems are causing the most difficulty and then tries to find ways to address those problems.

In some circumstances you may:

- agree to visit the patient at home or outside the hospital, e.g. in a café. This should be rare but might be necessary to re-engage the patient in treatment.
- offer telephone contact outside a crisis on a limited basis. This is more usual, particularly if a patient does not attend. After nonattendance at a session the patient should be contacted on the telephone. We have already mentioned that phone contact may also be made in response to positive developments as well.

The clinician needs to be assiduous about following up patients who do not attend appointments. Nonattendance breaks the clinician–patient agreement and needs exploration. At the beginning of treatment patients are given the telephone number to call in the event of a crisis and this number can be used if they cannot attend sessions. It is useful if the unit telephones have an answering machine and response times within working hours of the clinician are agreed and documented. Outside working hours the patient is asked to use the normal emergency system. Telephone discussions should be short and focused on the immediate problem.

Motivation

Enhancing a patient's motivation for treatment is part of the initial process of engaging a patient in treatment (Miller & Rollnick, 2002). All mental health professionals are able to use some motivational interviewing techniques.

Exploring what the patient expects to get out of treatment, identifying the risks of treatment, and considering the possible outcome of not engaging in treatment are all key areas to cover in the initial meetings. They are important when identifying the primary therapeutic aims with the patient and when discussing the emerging formulation. Equally important is identifying problems that might arise in treatment and specifying these whenever possible.

Ambivalence to treatment is an inevitable consequence of the patient's previous experience of health services and a natural uncertainty about changing the status quo, however unstable that might be. Some patients find it helpful to use the scales or balance sheet analogy. On one side of the scales there are two weights: the costs of maintaining things as they are and the benefits of change. The patient considers a change in each one and what effect that has on the balance of the scales. There may be a number of costs or benefits dependent on a single behavior. For example, the cost of continuing to self-harm might be being unable to wear short sleeves whereas the cost of change might be feeling increasingly angry, the benefit of stopping self-harm might be feeling better about oneself, which needs balancing with the anger, and the benefit of continuing to self-harm is that a relationship continues. The clinician helps the patient draw this out pictorially, discussing and agreeing on the changing balance of the scales.

Addressing the motivation of the patient is an initial step in developing a therapeutic alliance, a concept we have discussed in Chapter 2 and we now consider it further in relation to general treatment strategies.

Therapeutic alliance

In our original manual outlining SCM for BPD we suggested that the therapeutic alliance has three primary components:

- relationship or bond between clinician and client
- joint understanding of the techniques/methods employed in the therapy
- agreement regarding the goals of therapy.

We emphasized the importance of focusing on these aspects throughout therapy for good reason. Gunderson and colleagues (Gunderson, Najavits, & Leonhard et al., 1997) found that ratings of the alliance by clinicians treating patients with BPD were predictive of subsequent drop-out. Lingiardi et al. (2005) showed that early therapeutic alliance evaluations are good predictors of drop-out when treating people with personality disorders and that clinicians evaluate alliances with patients with BPD as significantly more negative when compared to ratings they give when treating patients with other personality disorders. In BPD the level of interpersonal sensitivity of the patient is high, which may affect the sensitivity of the clinician who, feeling criticized, undervalued, lacking in skills, and ineffective, rates the alliance low. This feasibly translates into premature conclusions in the mind of clinicians that they do not have the skills to treat the patients.

The alliance is a continuously oscillating relationship that can be affected by both patient and clinician, hence the importance of keeping it in mind throughout treatment. The ability of the clinician to repair ruptures in the alliance is crucial (Safran & Muran, 2000) and this requires attention to the relationship between the clinician and the patient.

Developing a positive alliance early in therapy is one of the primary aims of the clinician (Martin, 2000). There are some clinician factors that will increase the likelihood of developing a positive alliance and some factors that might decrease the possibility of forming a working agreement. Flexibility, respect, openness, and being interested are obvious components of any therapeutic relationship. Without experiencing these attitudes from the clinician, the patient will not be able to engage in meaningful treatment. The therapeutic alliance will be enhanced if the clinician avoids being rigid, distant, secretive, and inappropriately silent.

- Listen to the client's concerns in a manner which is nonjudgmental, supportive, and sensitive.
- Ensure that the client is clear about the rationale for the intervention being offered.
- Answer any questions about treatment in a straightforward manner.
- Respond to concerns openly and nondefensively in order to resolve any ambiguities.
- Help the patient express any concerns they have about the therapy and/or the clinician, especially when this relates to mistrust or skepticism.

Maintaining a therapeutic alliance

Patients with BPD are known to have negative responses to therapy, particularly if they feel they are not being taken seriously and are being misunderstood. It is important that, when implementing SCM, a negative response from the patient is seen as an opportunity to develop the relationship rather than an occasion to end the treatment. If there is a rupture in the alliance the clinician will:

- revisit the rationale for treatment and review this
- seek out any misunderstandings in therapy and clarify them
- refocus on tasks and goals which are seen as relevant to the patient.

Substance abuse

We mentioned in Chapter 1 the frequent co-occurrence of drug and alcohol abuse and even addiction in patients with BPD. Trull and coworkers reviewed the empirical literature between 1987 and 1997 on the comorbidity between BPD and substance use disorders. They found 17 studies that provided comorbidity rates of substance abuse in individuals diagnosed as BPD and 26 studies that provided comorbidity rates of BPD in individuals with substance abuse. Among BPD participants, 57.4% received a substance abuse diagnosis. More specifically, 48.8% in this group met criteria for an alcohol use disorder, while 38.0% had a drug use disorder. The prevalence of BPD among individuals with substance abuse were as follows: 27.4% had BPD among those with unspecified substance abuse, 14.3% had BPD among those with alcohol abuse/dependence, 16.8% had BPD among those with cocaine abuse/dependence, and 18.8% had BPD among those with opioid abuse/dependence. An intriguing question is whether BPD leads to substance abuse or drug problems cause subsequent symptoms of BPD. Patients often state that they only use drugs to manage their feelings and if they felt better and more stable they would not use drugs. This question was partially addressed but not answered in a longitudinal study of a random sample of children from upstate New York, who were assessed for Axis I and Axis II disorder first in 1983 at mean age 13.7 (2.6 SD), and most recently in follow-up at mean age 33.2 (2.9 SD). The study revealed that several personality disorders, schizotypal, borderline, narcissistic, and passive-aggressive, as well as conduct disorder, which precedes adult antisocial disorder, in early adolescence were significantly related to later substance abuse disorders (Cohen, Chena, Crawford, Brook, & Gordon, 2007). But whatever the cause of the comorbidity, the SCM clinician needs to assess the level of substance abuse right from the start and take a decision about involving appropriate services if necessary. Certainly patients who are harmfully physiologically addicted need referral for specialist help; those who use drugs and alcohol to manage their emotions but are not physiologically addicted require some psychoeducation about drugs and alcohol. This can be done in the problem-solving group. But the clinician implementing SCM initially outlines the dangers of drug misuse not only to physical health but also to the treatment response. A patient who smokes cannabis on a daily basis is unlikely to respond to treatment as well as someone who does not use drugs. The data from the trial of MBT versus SCM suggest that the positive effects of both treatments are reduced by use of substances but the reduction is greater in SCM.

The clinician will ask regularly about substance misuse in sessions and use similar techniques to those used for tackling self-harm (see the section on self-harm in Chapter 4) to reduce reliance on unprescribed drugs.

Stabilizing medication

In Chapter 1 we pointed out that most patients with BPD are offered medication and that the majority take the prescribed drugs, albeit often irregularly, in a desperate attempt to reduce their distress. Consequently SCM provides an opportunity for the patient to discuss medication. The use of medication is discussed in detail in Chapter 86. In sum, regular meetings with a psychiatrist should be integrated into the treatment plan and we suggest the patient is given medication review appointments on a 3–4 monthly basis, with the proviso that either the clinician or patient can request an earlier appointment. The primary clinician will liaise with the psychiatrist before and after each appointment but more importantly will discuss with the patient before the appointment how she is going to use the meeting and afterwards review how it unfolded.

There are a number of questions that prescribers and the primary clinician need to ask themselves (Tyrer & Bateman, 2004). These self-reflective questions include:

+ Do you need to revisit the treatment plan rather than change medication?
+ Can you avoid using medication if you implement an appropriate psychological or other intervention?
+ Are you cogniscent of only using a single drug wherever possible and avoiding polypharmacy?
+ Have you reflected on the influence of your relationship with the patient on your prescribing decisions?
+ Are you sure that you are not prescribing as a result of professional anxiety?

Comprehensive formulation

The formulation arises out of the comprehensive assessment. The assessment will include a detailed history of the patient's life and their symptoms: the history of the current problems, past psychiatric and forensic history, past medical history, personal and family history, and a detailed outline of impulsive behavior and suicide and self-harm attempts. To develop a formulation for SCM the clinician needs not only to obtain a general idea of the nature of the client's problem but also to generate an understanding about the patient's attitude and motivation for therapy. To do so the patient and clinician will:

+ appraise the benefits and disadvantages of engaging in therapy for the patient; help the patient recognize positive factors and possible dangers
+ acknowledge factors that might interfere with engaging in therapy—include practical issues, e.g. child care and transport, as well as motivational factors

- identify current stressors and personal and environmental factors provoking stress
- work to define current helpful coping mechanisms and to consider unhelpful responses to stress
- identify/select target symptoms or problems and consider which are the most distressing and which the most amenable to intervention
- help the client translate vague/abstract complaints into more concrete and discrete problems.

The formulation links motivational factors, symptom profiles, and interpersonal problems to treatment plans. Finally, a set of target areas are listed in order of current importance and agreed whenever possible between both patient and clinician. Where there is disagreement this should be noted. For example, a patient, in contrast to the clinician, may not consider repeated self-harm as being important.

Explanation of treatment approach

The patient has now completed an assessment, discussed the diagnosis, developed a crisis plan, identified risk factors, established a hierarchy of treatment aims, understood patient and clinician responsibilities, identified their level of motivation for treatment, and worked on a formulation of problems. It remains for the clinician to discuss the treatment approach. No patient with BPD should start treatment without understanding the focus of that treatment and how it might help her get better.

There are two therapy components to SCM, an individual meeting and a group meeting. Both aspects of the treatment focus specifically on the problem areas established collaboratively with the patient. A number of general therapy techniques are used and an outline of these forms the core of Chapter 3. In addition, resource-efficient treatment strategies are deployed (see Chapter 8) and many of these can be discussed with the patient at this point.

The clinician's explanation of treatment focuses on how treatment will (a) offer support, (b) help the patient find solutions to external problems, (c) provide some advocacy on their behalf at times, (d) seek to aid them manage emotional states, and (e) explore what to do to improve relationships. At no point will the clinician say that they have the answers; the clinician indicates that the work is about finding the answers.

Families, relatives, partners, and others

SCM involves families, relatives, partners, and others closely involved with the patient at this point in the pathway to treatment. Although we made no formal requirement for the SCM clinician to see families and others, it is part of good practice to at least inform people closely involved with the patient about what is happening. Explanation of the treatment approach for families can be helpful simply because the family may support the patient to attend treatment (Gunderson, 2008). It may also allow the family to have a better understanding of the disorder itself, potentially enabling them to be more responsive and constructive in their responses. Chapter 8 is devoted to working with families and friends.

Chapter 4

Structured clinical management: core treatment strategies

Summary

Core treatment strategies focus on key symptom areas of BPD:

+ emotion management
+ mood regulation
+ impulse control
+ interpersonal sensitivity
+ interpersonal problems
+ suicidality and self-harm.

Interventions can be categorized as nonspecific and specific and are summarized in Table 4.1. Both are equally important and are combined by the generalist clinician into a coherent therapeutic process.

Patient and clinician define target problems in individual sessions and map them against five modules which are organized around the key symptom areas of BPD and delivered in a problem-solving group.

The problem-solving group is used to work on the problem areas using patient-specific examples whenever possible. Strategies are developed in the group to help members to:

+ tolerate emotions
+ manage mood changes
+ control impulses
+ reduce self-harm
+ monitor sensitivity in interpersonal interaction.

In the previous chapter we outlined general treatment strategies, emphasizing the structure and organization of treatment and the care pathway along which the patient enters treatment. We now turn to some of the therapeutic

Table 4.1 Types of interventions

Nonspecific interventions	Specific interventions
Interviewing skills	Tolerating emotions
Attitude	Mood regulation
Empathy	Impulse control
Validation	Self-harm
Positive regard	Sensitivity and interpersonal problems
Advocacy	

interventions the clinician uses for treatment itself. The principles underpinning interventions used in SCM are that they have to be within the competence of the generalist mental health clinician without requiring extensive additional training and they have to focus on the symptom areas of BPD, namely emotion management, mood regulation, impulse control, interpersonal sensitivity, self-harm, and interpersonal problems. Further, the interventions can be divided into nonspecific and specific techniques (see Table 4.1).

The program itself combines individual sessions with a problem-solving group. Both the nonspecific and the specific interventions are used in the individual meetings. The work in the problem-solving group, an open group (patients joining at any time) and lasting for 1.5 hours, is organized around modules focusing on the specific interventions listed above.

Nonspecific interventions

Interviewing

Basic interviewing skills used by clinicians in their everyday practice form the foundation on which other interventions rest. *Open questions* are important—those that invite expansion of the topic rather than factual statements.

> *"You were telling me about lots of problems—is there one that you would like to discuss first?"*
> *"What made you pick that topic in particular?"*
> *"What do you make of that?"*

As the patient answers, the clinician *listens attentively* and reflects on what is being said. Demonstrating a questioning attitude as well as showing acceptance about how the patient feels is a skilful balancing act. In order to maintain this stance the clinician avoids making statements that chide the patient, stimulate argument or criticize her viewpoint, and refrains from rapidly providing a solution to the problem. To do so will more likely result in the patient closing down rather than opening up, and being told by the patient that the suggested solution has already been tried and failed. The clinician's task is to facilitate a process in which patients feel more secure about talking about themselves and working on their own solutions.

At times the clinician needs to actively *reinforce positive aspects* of how the patient manages and directly affirms her efforts by giving compliments and congratulating her on how she has coped. In doing so it is important to identify the "how" of the coping so that it can be carefully defined and repeated. Clinicians need to be aware that occasionally for some patients praise is not reinforcing, rather decreasing the likelihood of the behavior occurring again. In this situation the clinician will need to look for a reinforce other than praise that applies to the specific patient.

Finally you will want *to clarify and to summarize* carefully what the patient has been saying. This will demonstrate that you have been listening and potentially generate a feeling in the patient that things are being understood.

The hasty patient

Patient:I broke up with my boyfriend last week. I have had enough.

Therapist:Tell me more about what happened.

Patient:We were talking and his phone went off and he looked at it and turned it off a bit too quickly. I asked him who it was and he would not tell me. I tried to grab it off him to see who it was.

Therapist:Describe what you were feeling at the time.

Patient:I felt that he was seeing someone else and that he didn't want me to know about it.

Therapist:So, to clarify, his quickly turning off his phone led you becoming a bit suspicious. Is that right?

Patient:Yes.

Clinician attitude

The attitude of the clinician is vital to effective management of patients with BPD. In Chapter 2 we discussed some of the temperamental characteristics of clinicians who work successfully with people with BPD, exemplified by intrinsic patience, compassion, sensitivity, and robust sense of self. It is not easy to train others in these very personal characteristics but a number of other factors, which are responsive to training, are equally essential. Clinicians must have an enthusiasm for the work, a willingness to work in a team, an ability to maintain hope in the face of adversity, a capability to focus on the patient's subjective experience, and, most importantly, an inquisitive and curious attitude. These attitudes of the clinician may be developed and supported through training and team strategies.

Authenticity and openness

Authenticity of the clinician is promoted as a desirable characteristic in all the evidence-based manuals developed for use in generalist psychiatric services. It is essential that a patient experiences "a person" in front of them, someone who reacts and shows natural responsiveness. In training we have called this "putting the human back into the clinician"—"ask yourself what you would say to a friend who was telling you this story?" The inactive, nonresponsive, silently observing clinician engenders terror in patients with BPD. This can inadvertently result in harm. Equally an overly active clinician, who provides solutions prematurely, "has all the answers," and "knows everything," will fail to generate the patient's own capability and risks undermining developing abilities of self-reliance. A balance of activity is required.

BPD patients characteristically are sensitive to external cues such as facial expressions (Lynch et al., 2006) and body movements, and make rapid assumptions from this information about the clinician's underlying thoughts and feelings. These assumptions may be accurate, partially accurate or, as with most people, at times, frankly wrong. It is important to emphasize that people with BPD are as accurate as the general population in identifying facial expression except when the expression is neutral, when the person with BPD is more likely to interpret it as having a higher level of threat (Fertuck et al., 2009). It is especially important that therapists do not deny a patient's accurate perception of their facial expression, which is inherently invalidating and can only serve to fuel the doubt the patient has about their own experience. As Glenn Gabbard stated: "neutrality is dead."

Two components of SCM counter the tendency for people with BPD to interpret threat in the context of neutral facial expression whilst simultaneously promoting an active transparent therapist.

First, the clinician is advised to make his current mental processes about the patient transparent, openly deliberating when possible. Returning to the "hasty patient":

Patient:You are not interested in what I am saying are you?
Therapist:Actually you have picked up on something. My mind was still caught on what we were talking about before. I was still thinking about what happened with your boyfriend. I don't quite understand how the speed of his reaction links to him seeing someone else.

This sort of answer requires a directness, honesty, authenticity, and personal ownership, which is problematic partly because of the dangers of boundary violations in the treatment of BPD. Our emphasis on the need for authenticity from the generalist mental health clinician is not a license to overstep ethical boundaries of therapy; we are merely stressing that the clinician needs to make himself mentally available to the patient and must demonstrate an ability to balance uncertainty and doubt with a continued struggle to understand. This becomes particularly important when patients correctly identify feelings and thoughts experienced by the clinician.

Second, the clinician develops a recurrent focus in the problem-solving group on the patient's sensitivity and assumptions about others and the evidence they use to understand others' intent (see section on sensitivity and interpersonal problems in Chapter 4 for a discussion of this focus).

The clinician needs to be prepared for questions that put him on the defensive—"You're bored with me," "You don't like me much either, do you?" etc. Such challenges to the clinician can arise suddenly and without warning and the clinician needs to be able to answer with authenticity. If he does not do so the patient will become more insistent and this might evoke the very experience he is complaining of; being told repeatedly you are irritated when you are not is likely to be experienced as irritating by most people.

A patient's accurate perception of what is in the clinician's mind needs validation (Bateman & Fonagy, 2006; Linehan, 1993a).

If the clinician is indeed feeling bored or irritated, it is important that he says so in a way that stimulates exploration of what is boring within the current patient–clinician interaction.

> *"Now you mention it, I was feeling a bit bored and I am unsure where that is coming from. Is it related to what you are talking about or how you are talking about it or is it more my problem at the moment? You know I am really not sure."*

If the clinician is not bored, then he needs to find a way to express this in a way that opens up the possibility of exploring what stimulated the patient's question. Do not reflect the question to the patient, "What makes you think that I am bored?," so often a favorite technique of the clinician who does not know what to do. This will annoy a patient with BPD, who will experience it as an evasion and not an invitation to explore themselves further.

A statement such as:

> *"As far as I am aware, I was not bored. In fact, I was trying to grasp what you were saying. I felt muddled. But now I am intrigued that you and I were having such a different experience of this at the moment. Was there something I was doing that made you think I was bored?"*

is far more likely to further the dialogue.

Knowing versus not-knowing

The clinician must accept that both he and his patient experience things only subjectively and that neither has primacy of knowledge about the other or about what has happened. This stance of the clinician is used specifically in mentalization-based treatment (Bateman & Fonagy, 2004, 2006) but also forms part of the therapist's general strategy in SCM, albeit with less methodical implementation. We see this stance as a basic way of interacting with people with BPD.

When did you as a clinician last say to a patient—"You *must* be feeling … ?" The use of the word "must" implies that you *know* what the patient is feeling, even if the patient has not expressed the feeling. Of course, you might be correct about the feeling of the patient but equally you might be wrong. Our own representation of a feeling can never be the same as that of our patients. The problem in treatment of BPD is that our patients will all too readily agree with our suggestions, taking them on.

A common confusion has been that being a not-knowing clinician is equivalent to feigning ignorance and that knowing is telling the patient what to do. Nothing could be further from the truth. The clinician has a mind and has had experience in life and is well trained. But he is not an expert on the mental processes of the patient. So he continually demonstrates that he can use his mind and has learned from experience. He may hold alternative perspectives to the patient and, if he does, this provides the perfect opportunity for further exploration.

The beauty of the not-knowing stance is that it reminds the clinician that they do not need to understand what the patient is saying or to struggle to make sense of it within another framework such as the patient's traumatic past or their underlying cognitive schemas. Indeed it means that the clinician does not have to have the solution. What the clinician does have though, is the knowledge about how to work out solutions. Relieved of having to understand, the novice clinician is in a more confident position. It allows him to be less fearful of making errors.

Clinician error

All clinicians sometimes get things wrong. We say something inappropriate, we forget sessions, we fail to fulfill promises, we persistently do not understand something the patient is telling us. We need to be aware of what should be done when something goes wrong and be able to explore what has happened that led to the error. Clearly, clinician errors range from the mild to the severe, but all offer an opportunity to revisit what happened and to learn more about context, experience, and feelings engendered in both patient and clinician as a result of the error. Importantly, as clinicians we take initial responsibility for our part in what happens when something goes wrong in a session. We balance reference to our own responsibility for something that has happened with stimulating a process in which the patient's contribution can also be explored if it is relevant. An excessive emphasis on the patient's share of the responsibility will alienate her. Patients with BPD feel, understandably, that they are blamed for most things. As soon as the patient feels that they are being made to feel that "everything is their fault" they are likely either to withdraw or attack. So we always start from the perspective that we, rather than the patient, have done something wrong.

The misunderstanding therapist

Patient: I can't believe that you said that. If you think that about me then it means you have no understanding of me at all.

Therapist: What was it that I said that was so off the mark?

Patient: That's the point—if you have no idea it just shows that you have not been listening to me at all.

Therapist: I am sorry but I am not quite sure. I was mentioning that you seemed to have much stronger abilities to manage on your own.

Patient: But I have been talking about how much I need a girlfriend and how it is not OK to be on my own. Just because I manage does not mean that I don't need a partner.

Therapist: Oh I see. I am sorry about that I had not meant that just because you seemed to be happy on your own that we need not be concerned about difficulties in not having a partner.

Empathy

Clinicians use empathic responding in their daily work—we comment on what the patient is feeling to show that we share it in some way. For example, we might say when listening to a story from a patient about being ill-treated by a partner "that was so hurtful of them," "You seem to feel very hurt by the way you were treated." But empathy is more than this. It is a process whereby the clinician finds a way to experience and to perceive the reality of the patient and responds to this in a way that demonstrates that understanding. In empathy you show that you are following the patient's feelings and not imposing your reality. You need to be aware that the patient may be highly sensitive to your evaluation of their internal states. They value your opinion because they often find their own states of mind confusing.

Baron-Cohen (2008) has suggested that emotion understanding is based on self-affect propositions, by contrast to understanding others' thoughts, which is mediated by agent-attribute propositions. Thus, interpersonal emotion understanding invariably starts from a self-state. In contrast, to understand the other person's cognitive state we separate physical reality from mental reality ("agent-attribute propositions"). The proposition "John thinks it is raining" is true irrespective of the presence or absence of rain. By contrast, ascribing emotion is based on extending or generalizing from one's own experience ("self-affect-state propositions"). The clinician relies on his own affective understanding to be empathic and experiences an emotional state. There can be no empathy without this affective sharing because there has to be *interpersonal similarity* between the empathizer and the patient. This distinguishes empathy from sympathy. A sympathetic clinician does not experience, for example, empathetic rage whereas by definition the empathic clinician does. So we ask the mental health clinician to distinguish his sympathetic and empathic responses so that their meaning can be discussed in the team meetings. Finally it is important that, where relevant, the clinician remains aware that his feeling arises from the patient, even if he feels it empathically himself, and that he does not ascribe it to himself. A clinician may feel angry on behalf of a patient but does not enact that anger by taking up the cause of the patient. He will use his empathic understanding of the patient's anger to inform problem-solving, for example (see below).

The timid patient

A patient was talking about difficulties in her relationship, describing her boyfriend as someone who did not pay adequate attention to her and how it disturbed her. The clinician said "it is annoying feeling ignored and not knowing what to do about it." This is an empathic statement which tries to show the patient that the clinician is seeing it from the point of view of the patient. The patient said that she knew that she could not leave her boyfriend because she loved him. After she had talked about this a bit more, the clinician said "perhaps you worry about him leaving you if you try to talk to him about what is upsetting you." This was an attempt to abstract further from what the patient was saying and to deepen the empathic understanding. It allowed the patient to talk about her fears that if she made any demands on her boyfriend he would leave her.

Validation

Validation involves active observing, reflection, and direct validation. The first two aspects of validation are common to every therapy. Direct validation requires the therapist to take a nonjudgmental attitude, another essential aspect to all therapies, as we mentioned earlier, and search for the essential validity of the patient's experience and responses rather than its dysfunctional characteristics (Linehan, 1993a, 1997). Direct validation forms a crucial aspect of the interaction between the clinician and patient. It is used to confirm the patient's experience and contingent response as being understandable in a specific context. If a patient says "I am a fool," the task of the therapist is to find the truth in the statement. The kindly clinician is naturally more likely to try to oppose the self-criticism and reassure the patient. But reassuring the patient that he is not a fool is likely to be ineffective and simply result in him feeling misunderstood. Saying something like, "I totally get it that you have thoughts of being a fool, and you have never appeared a fool to me. Do tell me how you arrive at the thought that you are a fool at this moment" is both validating and offers a pathway to developing an alternative perspective.

When as clinicians we are stuck trying to find something to validate, we can always validate our clients' experience, and often can validate the severity of their distress, and the difficulty of change.

The hasty patient

Patient:I tried to grab the phone off him and he would not give it to me. That confirmed that he was hiding something so I said that I knew he was having an affair and he didn't want me to know about it. He said that I was being stupid. Well that did it. I went mad and threw my drink at him. What was I supposed to do?

Clinician:Well maybe we can have a think about that but first of all I can see that if you were so caught up in how you felt and were convinced at that moment that he was having an affair you had to do something (validating the valid aspects of the situation). What was it you were feeling?

Patient:I went mad.

Clinician:I meant more when he said that you were being stupid. That sounded as if it had been the final straw

Patient:He was ignoring what I felt.

Clinician:Saying you were stupid really sounds dismissive to me and most of us would be hurt by that—I know how sensitive you are to that.

Positive regard

Positive regard and respect for patients is a central aspect of the work of all mental health clinicians (Rogers, 1986). It is important that the clinician takes a nonjudgmental attitude to the patients, values their humanity, and recognizes their personal struggle. This is represented by responsiveness and warmth to the client.

Warmth needs to be conveyed in the context of a professional boundary. There are many ways to do this in behavior and verbal response:

+ shake hands with the patient when greeting them
+ smile

- use a warm tone of voice
- maintain eye contact
- inject humor
- genuine interest
- remain hopeful.

When the clinician is aware of feeling negative about a patient or, equally importantly, overly positive and protective, he must discuss this in supervision and implement the following procedure.

Write down answers to the following questions:

- What do I like about my patient and what are her positive features?
- What do I dislike about my patient and what are her negative features?
- Is there anything that I am aware of that might have brought about my current response?

Discuss your answers in the supervision session.

Advocacy

Advocacy work is inherently supportive and includes elements of the following:

- helping the patient plan how to deal with life problems in an effective way
- providing information about rights and structures of organizations that the patient is negotiating with (e.g., housing, probation)
- helping the patient write letters to or arrange appointments with any person, organization or authority who can offer support
- preparing the patient for meetings with, for example, social workers, psychiatrists, landlords, the police, probation
- making links with family and carers, community mental health teams, legal representatives and so on.

All this work will be done as part of case management but importantly you will follow it through carefully in the individual work with the patient. Rather than doing everything "for" the patient, the advocacy role involves the clinician adhering to some of the attitudes we have discussed earlier in this chapter and included encouraging the patient to do as much as possible themselves. At first sight the not-knowing stance of the clinician that we recommend may appear antipathetic to the advocacy role but in fact they complement each other by ensuring patients have the information and support they need to start working on how they take the issue forward for themselves.

Support in the context of your advocacy work is defined according to a number of components, which include:

+ active reassurance
+ explanation of difficulties in psychological and psychiatric terms
+ finding out information for the patient
+ guidance when a problem remains unsolved
+ suggestions about how to manage difficulties
+ encouragement about personal efficacy
+ permission to express feelings about others as well as oneself.

Specific interventions

Problem-solving skills in a group context

The group component of the program follows a problem-solving approach (Huband, McMurran, Evans, & Duggan, 2007). The group leader is "in charge" of the group. "In charge" is not used here to suggest that the group leader is autocratic but to imply that the group leader manages the group carefully to ensure that problems are covered adequately and are discussed in enough detail to ensure that all patients are aware of potential solutions. Hence we recommend the group leader stimulates and focuses the discussion as much as possible. Maintaining a balance between providing solutions on the one hand and developing solutions from the discussion of the patients on the other is a key skill for group leaders. The group leader should be careful not to be too lecturing or knowing in her style, as this tends to encourage passivity in the group members.

Practical problems

SCM uses an unashamedly practical problem-solving approach to find answers to patient difficulties. The target problems are defined in two ways. First, the clinician and patient define as many problems as possible in the assessment and these are considered further in the individual sessions and agreed between patient and clinician. These are then mapped against five areas of problems of BPD which form the five modules of the problem-solving group:

+ tolerance of emotions
+ mood regulation
+ impulse control
+ self-harm
+ sensitivity and interpersonal problems.

Second, problems may be identified in the problem-solving group and agreed between the clinician and the group members. Once the problem is defined it is broken down into small components, particularly if it is complex. Progressive steps are then developed which, when negotiated, have the potential to solve the problem. Subsequent work in the group focuses solely on progress with the problem-solving steps. For example, if four steps are identified, the clinician will ensure that each is taken in turn by the group and resolved before moving on to the next step. To achieve this, the clinician will:

- identify the problem—discuss this in the group and/or individual sessions and generate a hierarchy of problems
- agree on the first problem to be solved if there are a number
- discuss steps towards achieving a solution to the problem—brainstorm solutions
- share their own possible solutions to the problem but remain neutral about whether the patient uses them or not
- assess advantages and disadvantages of all the solutions suggested
- ask the patients to report back the following week on the results
- revisit the solutions to see if they can be improved.

A patient stated that his problem was getting repairs done to his accommodation by the local authority, who were responsible for renovating his kitchen after a fire. When a plumber arrived at the flat he had none of the parts needed for the cooker and sink. The patient became angry and threatened him. The plumber left hurriedly and reported that it was unsafe for people to attend the flat unaccompanied by the police. How was the patient to get his repairs done and also assure the plumber and others that his outburst would not occur again? The clinician asked the group to consider the possible steps that the patient might take to achieve his aims. Initially there was some discussion about the patient's rights and how he might send a threatening letter, but it was recognized that this was unlikely to achieve his aim and might even impede a successful outcome. With help from the clinician the patients decided there were a number of steps. First, he had to make a list of everything that needed to be done. Second, he had to contact the council to apologize for what happened and ask how he could assure them that it was safe for people to visit without the police. Third, he had to be welcoming if someone attended. Fourth, he had to manage any feelings he had about the repair man.

It will be apparent that one aspect to the practical problem here is the patient's sensitivity in the interpersonal interaction. This indicates that, once the breakdown of the problem is complete, the clinician needs to invoke the module related to sensitivity and interpersonal problems. Similarly if the group agree that excessive anger is part of the difficulty, the module on tolerating emotions is invoked.

Symptoms of BPD

The axiom for the clinician is first define the problem and break it down into solvable components; second seek out the area(s) of BPD that have been activated by the context the patient is in. Then invoke the appropriate module. This problem-solving analysis is followed both in the individual sessions and in the group work.

To reiterate, in SCM, problems that patients bring are placed, whenever possible, into the five categories:

- tolerance of emotions
- mood regulation
- impulse control
- self-harm
- sensitivity and interpersonal problems.

In this section we cover the basic problem-solving strategies that can help patients with BPD achieve a reduction in their symptoms. Detail about complementary and overlapping strategies, for example chain analysis, are discussed in Chapter 8. The techniques described here were used in SCM delivered in the randomized controlled trial. They are easily learned and can be implemented by generalist mental health professionals with brief training. Some of those we consider as resource-efficient strategies (see Chapter 8) may require more training and practice.

Each problem area described here should be considered as a treatment "module." Problem-solving groups, at the beginning of treatment, focus on each of them in turn, devoting the whole group or a series of groups to each topic.

Once the clinician has covered all modules, he is at liberty to vary the topic of the group but must continually return to the modules when indicated. As we have already mentioned, the primary indicator to use a module is when a patient describes one of the problem areas. So if a patient reports self-harm the clinician insists on focusing on the event and works within the frame of the self-harm module. Similarly, if a patient talks about an impulsive action, the impulse control module is invoked.

Tolerance of emotions

Discussion of emotions is likely to lead to a discussion of mood and vice versa so this module may become mixed with the module on mood management, but whenever possible it is recommended that the clinician focuses on them separately.

Time spent on how to manage different feelings forms a specific focus of this module. Patients with BPD have feelings like all of us but often experience them as more powerful than other individuals; they find them more easily triggered. They cannot return to their baseline emotion easily and the strength of their emotions often results in them taking action to reduce their distress and/or the experience that their emotions are controlling them. Sometimes patients close off experiencing emotions because they are afraid of their emotions. Sometimes patients want "not to feel" and ask us how to stop feeling. Don't be fooled by this; our task is to help our patients to continue to experience their emotions but not to feel overcome by them.

Write this on the flip chart—"How can I have feelings and manage them without harmful action?"

> The clinician asks the patients to identify common feelings and also to note those that they find a problem.

A number of feelings are commonly described, including shame, anger, frustration, entitlement, fear, anxiety, and misery. It is noteworthy that patients often only come up with displeasing emotions and yet they may also find feelings of love, affection, sincerity, curiosity, for example, an equal problem. It is sensible for the clinician to note this and to ensure some of the more pleasing emotions are also identified.

The clinician can give information about emotions to focus the discussion and we repeat here some of the aspects of emotions that patients have found useful and are currently used in a mentalization-based therapy psychoeducational program (Karterud & Bateman, 2011).

When the identification of emotions is reasonably complete, the clinician suggests that emotions can be categorized in various ways. Some people divide emotions into basic emotions, which are present in all mammals, and social emotions, which only occur in higher primates and humans. Others talk about primary and secondary emotions, which overlap partly with basic emotions and social emotions, respectively. For example, a basic or primary emotion of anger may result in a belief about anger (e.g., I should not be angry), leading to a social or secondary emotion of shame.

> The clinician asks the patients to discuss basic emotions and social emotions, giving examples from their own lives.

The clinician summarizes seven basic emotions (Panksepp, 1998), prefacing this with a warning that there is considerable argument about the emotions that are best included:

1) interest and curiosity, exploratory behavior

2) fear

3) anger

4) sexual

5) separation anxiety/sadness

6) love/caring

7) play/joy.

These emotions can cause problems for all of us. Each serves a different biological function and can be adaptive. Normalizing emotions is usually experienced by patients as helpful.

The clinician emphasizes that some people differentiate between emotions and feelings. Emotions are at core the person's intrinsic bodily reaction, for example when our brains appraise something as dangerous this stimulates bodily symptoms. Feelings are the conscious experience of the body state during emotional activation. The clinician explains that because of their upbringing and socialization, people can be distanced from their natural, emotional reactions as well as being oversensitive to their power. This means that on the one hand some people react emotionally, but without necessarily feeling their emotions; on the other hand others are rapidly overcome by awareness of the intensity of their emotions and cannot resist their biological drive. There is danger in both responses. We can be emotionally activated unaware of what emotions are involved, and so unable to manage the emotion; or so overcome with the intensity of the feeling that actions are ill-considered at best and self-destructive at worst.

Primary and secondary emotions

Some authors make a distinction between primary and secondary emotions (Greenberg & Safran, 1987).

A primary emotion is an emotion that we experience in response to an internal or external event. A secondary emotion is an emotion we can have about the primary emotion on the basis of our self-critical beliefs about the primary emotion.

For example, anxiety about attending a job interview is a primary emotion. If we then have a self-critical belief about our anxiety such as, "I should not be anxious" then it is likely that we will have additional feelings such as more anxiety, guilt, shame or sadness about the primary emotion of anxiety. We will now be anxious about being anxious or feel shame about being anxious or sad about being anxious. We can see how this will make the already challenging situation even harder. Not only do we have to deal with our primary anxiety we also have to deal with our secondary shame, guilt, sadness or anxiety.

Secondary emotions are often more problematic than primary emotions. This is because they are associated with self-critical self-beliefs, prevent us accessing our primary emotions, and confuse the picture when we are trying to identify our primary emotions.

The solution to the problem of secondary emotions is theoretically simple but challenging to do. The solution to getting rid of our secondary emotions is to be accepting of our primary emotions. To be less distressed by our emotions, we need to be more welcoming and accepting of our primary emotions whatever they are. This includes not only emotions that are pleasurable but also those that are distressing, including sadness, anxiety, and anger. If we are able to do this, and act skillfully whatever our primary emotion, we are then left with our primary emotions only, without the additional burden of our secondary emotions.

Consumer comment

I tried avoiding feeling a lot of the time. When I then felt something like being angry, sad or happy, I would give myself a hard time and feel guilty for feeling what I did. This made every emotion more distressing. Once I learned to be fully present in the moment, and accept how I felt, I was able to work on managing the primary emotion, and thereby gain some control of my emotional states.

A number of strategies are suggested by the clinician for managing emotional states. These include identifying and labeling emotions, reflecting upon but not necessarily reacting to current emotions, and taking opposite action or expressing a countervalent emotional state, where it is wise to do so.

Identifying and labeling

Many patients with BPD find it hard to say how they feel; feelings are often a jumble of different sensations. Identifying and naming emotions is important if they are to be regulated and this is discussed further in the module on mood (see section on mood regulation in Chapter 4). The patient is asked to pause and to attend to their emotion, consider what has stimulated the emotion, note the context in which the emotion occurs, and recognize the pressure to act whilst resisting action where this is wise to do.

Reflecting but not necessarily reacting

Patients are asked to discuss feelings that are particularly associated with a strong urge to act. Pleasurable as well as displeasing emotions may be used as examples. Feelings of love can be associated with a strong urge to act without reflection as much as anger, for example. We are all prone to emotional reactivity and can regret what we say and do. The focus in this discussion is on inhibiting reactions whilst promoting reflection prior to taking any action. The aim is not to prevent actions but to ensure that actions are measured, appropriate to the situation, and are representative of the feeling. Too often feelings are taken as facts.

Opposite action/countervalent expression

Inappropriate or disproportionate responses to emotions, especially in interpersonal interactions, can be moderated by taking opposite action or expressing an emotion that runs counter to the emotion. For example, a feeling of anger could be moderated by doing something nice for the person or by expressing friendliness in the immediate context of the anger. This is not to suggest that feelings are suppressed, rather to manage relevant actions and/or strength of the feeling. It is important to emphasize this to prevent patients thinking that they should suppress feelings altogether.

Strategies

Engage the patients in identifying contexts in which individual group members find the intensity of their emotions leads to actions that they regret.

> The clinician asks members of the group to describe a recent situation when they have had strong reactions to an emotion.

- ◆ Work with the group to see if there are common situations that lead to strong emotions. Many of the contexts will be interpersonal and this is an area on which you can focus in the group.

Many situations that are described relate to feeling fearful, angry or ill-treated. It is important to determine if these feelings are primary or secondary before working further on them. Only primary experiences are considered at this point in the group. Once the emotion has been defined the group members are asked to think about techniques that might be helpful to reduce the inevitable reaction that follows.

> The clinician asks the group to outline ways in which they have been able to act skillfully despite the intense experience of emotion.

Initially it is useful to suggest that many techniques will be ways of reducing physiological tension as the basic emotions are felt within changes in the body, for example fearfulness and anxiety are signaled by a change in heart rate, sweating, feeling short of breath, as well as suddenly becoming vigilant and wary mentally. Managing these body sensations of overarousal takes precedence over developing ways to cope with interpersonal sensitivity. The clinician can inform the group that interpersonal sensitivity will be discussed at a later stage in the group itself or in a subsequent group.

- ◆ Discuss relaxation techniques for patients to use.
  - Progressive muscle relaxation.
  - Breathing skills.
  - Silence and meditation stance.
  - Yoga and holding postures.

These techniques are to be practiced in the group. Many patients find this useful and it is necessary for the clinician to return again and again to the practice of relaxation in the group and to do so at times of tension in the group itself. The clinician needs to be comfortable with running brief relaxation exercises and be able to motivate the patients to practice at home.

- ◆ Provide other basic strategies used for anxiety.
  - Distraction by engaging in other activities—Clinicians teach that distraction by definition avoids emotion experiencing and so should be used as little as possible, but used as much as necessary to prevent a destructive downward spiral.
  - Recognizing that anxiety can arise from automatic thoughts—if an emotion occurs the patients are asked to consider the associated feeling as a stimulus to thinking about what they are feeling—'What am I thinking right now or just before I had this feeling?'
  - Provide the patients with a daily thought record sheet if you think this will be helpful.

The clinician takes each basic strategy and discusses it in detail. For example:

The clinician asks what sort of distraction strategies people use.

List the activities that patients bring, for example going for a walk, leaving a situation, reading or doing jigsaw puzzles. Break this down into components, as the group will need to problem-solve the fact that in a crisis it can be very difficult to implement a complex strategy.

> How do we make sure we have the best chance to engage in distraction?

Work out with the patients how quickly this strategy can be implemented and whether it needs preparation between episodes of emotional difficulties. Discuss whether patients need to be often implementing distraction so that their feelings are not so easily provoked or if this is something to do when they are alerted to the danger. Again we want to maximize emotion tolerance by encouraging the limited use of distraction, saving distraction for occasions when not distracting will lead to an acute downward spiral.

The clinician needs to be aware that there are some patients with BPD, primarily those with marked interpersonal sensitivity, who find some relaxation exercises threatening. These individuals can feel that the clinician is trying to control them, to take over their mind, and they may refuse to engage in the exercises. For some patients, relaxation strategies inadvertently increase anxiety by decreasing their sense of self-control. This must be respected and work done with them to discover alternative ways of managing anxiety. This can be difficult as they often dismiss efforts to manage anxiety and fearfulness, and may do so in the group, saying that nothing works.

Mood regulation

The aim of managing emotions is to ensure that patients can have strong intense emotions and continue to act skillfully; that is, experience emotions and engage in skilful non-mood dependent behavior. But there is an additional problem, namely that some moods form the background to the patient's everyday life and are persistent. This state is painful and has to be addressed.

We have given some information about the co-occurrence of other disorders in BPD in Chapter 1. For this module it is important that the clinician is aware of this information and so we summarize the research a little further here. In most research studies the commonest co-occurring disorder is depression. Skodol et al. (2002) reviewed 16 studies where structured or semistructured diagnostic instruments were used to establish comorbidity. The findings are consistent. In a series of 409 nonpsychotic outpatients, 59 were diagnosed with BPD. Only one of these did not have a concurrent Axis I diagnosis and over two-thirds had three or more Axis I diagnoses (Zimmerman & Mattia, 1999). Sixty-one percent were diagnosed with major depressive disorder while 29% had panic disorder with agoraphobia and 13% substance misuse. In the biggest study of subjects with BPD comprehensively assessed for Axis I and Axis II disorders using both semistructured interviews and self-rating scales, of 501 patients, 240 were diagnosed with BPD (Skodol et al., 1999). Almost 40% of the BPD cases met criteria for at least one mood disorder. Thirty-one percent had major depression, 16% had dysthymia, 9% had bipolar-I, and 4% had bipolar-II.

Comorbidity may be an artifact of overlapping symptom sets used to define co-occurring disorders. Criteria for BPD include affective instability and recurrent suicidal threats or behaviors, both of which overlap with symptoms of major depressive disorder. The alternative hypothesis is that borderline and other Cluster B symptomatology is a complication that arises from a primary affective disorder (Akiskal, Hirschfeld, & Yerevanian, 1983). Thus, interpersonal maladjustment may be a residue of depressive illness, and chronic personality disorder may result from recurrent depressive episodes. On balance this explanation probably has the least evidence. Whichever account has the most merit, the co-occurrence of BPD and depressive symptoms is outlined to the group by the clinician at the start of working on depression and anxiety.

In terms of helping patients with BPD manage their emotions and moods and problem-solve we recommend linking their depression, sadness and other emotions to interpersonal interaction. SCM facilitates the processing of emotions by the patient acknowledging that emotional levels become too high (e.g., anger, fear, despair) or too low (e.g., apathy, low motivation). This causes patients problems in their interpersonal life so the therapist will:

- help the patient define his emotions and experience them in a way that facilitates change (see above "identifying and labeling emotions")
- explore the emotions in relation to the patient's relationships.

The clinician may wish to outline the importance that attachment to others plays in how we manage our emotions. As children we establish an attachment relationship to our caregivers and respond with separation anxiety when they leave us and then with sadness when the person does not return when expected. We suggest that this is one way of understanding our emotion and mood-related reactions, exemplified by our distress when a partner does not return a phone call soon enough. Psychodynamic theory names separation anxiety as a natural part of a type of protest phase connected to crying and screaming, which are used to attract attention to our plight. Sadness belongs to a later phase in which the protest has not had the desired result. The person is sad and low in mood, tired and with low self-esteem and has ruminative thoughts. She feels there is something wrong with her and secondary emotions arise. The person often has difficulties with concentrating, life seems meaningless and there seems to be little hope for the future. The thought of giving up on life may not be far away. In many people, these emotions pass but when the emotion remains intense for a longer time it organizes into a depressed mood with a background of anxiety. It is also normative to experience sadness when our desires for affiliation are greater than the person we wish to affiliate with is able or willing to match or when circumstances do not pragmatically allow for our affiliation needs to be met.

Strategies

◆ Awareness of emotions as signals.

> The clinician asks the group to consider the idea that emotions are an alert. What is an emotion telling us?

Emotions tell us to look around within and without ourselves—what is occurring in the immediacy of the moment, often in our current interaction with someone, what is happening in our life, what is going on in our mind at the time?

◆ Working out the events leading to emotions (see chain analysis for self-harm, p. 111).

> The clinician asks the patients for examples of an emotion in the same way as the emotions module. Take a range of emotions, preferably from a number of the patients in the group, but now engage them in working on surrounding events and context that might link to the emotion.

A more structured chain analysis is discussed in more detail in working with episodes of self-harm (p. 111) and in chapter 8. Often patients discover that the emotion that they have is normative and that most people would have a similar emotion given the context or situation. At times though a patient cannot easily identify and label an emotion with finesse (e.g., disgust, repulsion, anger vs awful, horrible, ugh). When this occurs the clinician engages the patients in a process of labeling emotions with precision—"If this was me I would feel angry, what would others think they would feel?"

> Can you try to describe the emotion in more detail and perhaps someone can help give it a name?

Labeling emotions is important and some of our clinicians give patients a list of emotions to illustrate the range of emotions that are known to occur. One patient stuck on his fridge a list of emotions, organized around groupings (e.g., sad, happy, angry). Whenever he was feeling something he could not easily label he looked down the list and tried to attach a name to it.

The same thing can be done with face cartoons demonstrating a wide range of emotions that patients can scroll through as they attempt to put a label to their experience.

A patient felt dismissed when someone she had just met stopped talking to her at a party and started conversing with someone else. She tapped him on the shoulder and said "Don't start ignoring me, I haven't finished what I was saying." He was rather taken aback. Shortly after, she got drunk and felt acutely depressed saying that she always felt like this really but at times it was covered up. Taking this example, the group, following the lead from the clinician, deconstructed the events, asking questions about the patient's experience of the other person before this event and exploring her feelings for him. What sort of person was he? What was it about him that you liked? It turned out that the feeling of being dismissed was actually something she was sensitive to, particularly at times when she liked someone. She easily felt that the person she liked did not take enough interest in her. So liking someone was identified as a vulnerability for her, which might lead to sadness. She said that she didn't want to stop liking people and so what was she supposed to do? This is the next problem to be tackled by the group—how do we manage a feeling of liking someone? The module of managing emotions is then followed.

Impulse control

We discussed the construct of impulsivity in Chapter 3 (see section on impulsivity). The aim of this module is to help the patient place a distance between triggering events and action. Write this aim on a flip chart.

The clinician outlines three major problem aspects of impulsivity:

- not attending: decreased attention—easily getting bored, inability to concentrate on a task, difficulty keeping to topic when something else comes into the mind

- not planning—lack of premeditation; limited consideration about or concern for consequences; excitement about risky activities that precludes considering negative consequences

- action: action without reflection—going into action rapidly, acting rashly sometimes related to pleasing as well as displeasing emotions.

> The clinician asks group members to describe some of their impulsive action urges and actions, come to an agreement about which ones they share in common, and describe how the three major problem aspects of impulsivity (attention, planning, action) manifest themselves—accepting that some actions will have aspects of all groupings.

Table 4.2 Impulsivity chart with example

Category	Emotion name	Urge	Indicators	Helpful response
Not attending	Boredom	Do something exciting	Awareness of inability to concentrate	Skilful action with others
Not planning	Anticipated satisfaction	Opportunistic theft	Awareness of thoughts of entitlement	Stop, think
Action	Loneliness	Find boyfriend, get drunk	Noticing action urge	Meet friends

Impulses that often arise in discussion, and may be given as examples by the clinician if patients are initially reluctant to share, are urges to contact a partner who does not return a call quickly enough, and engaging in reckless behavior, including sexual activity, excessive spending, and binge eating. The clinician and patients identify a few, usually no more than three (one action urge for each dominant problem category), that the majority of patients find relevant and write them in a box on the flip chart using the template in Table 4.2, in which an example is given. The clinician is primarily trying to engage the patients in a process of breaking down damaging impulsive events into component parts.

Strategies

◆ Name the impulse.

> The clinician asks the patients to describe an episode related to one of the aspects of impulsivity outlined earlier. Identify the action urge. Have there been any occasions when one of them has managed not to take action and, if so, how was this done?

- Discuss what an impulse is and explore ways in which each patient manages not to take action immediately. Go around the group asking each patient in turn. Write the answers down in the box on the template.

◆ Become aware of the indicators of likely action.

> The clinician asks the patients to identify what tells them they are likely to take action

- Consider bodily experiences, e.g. heart rate, breathing, flushing, stomach butterflies.
- Identify feelings, e.g. anger, upset, excitement, preparedness, vigilance.

◆ Slow down thoughts by observing and identifying each thought to generate a "long fuse."

> Now the clinician asks the patients to slow down their thoughts by observing and identifying each thought as they follow on from each other.

- Patients tend to jump rapidly to conclusions. Ask them to slow down and trace their thoughts. Ask them to identify any assumptions they make without checking out the facts.

◆ Self-monitor.

> The clinician asks the patients to now self-reflect. Are they acting on assumptions without checking out the facts? If a friend acted as they had done based on the assumption without checking out the facts what advice would they give?

- Do they notice that they are reacting rather than reflecting? If they discover that they would give alternative advice to a friend, the clinician can promote a wider discussion about the different advice that the group members identify.

> The clinician steers the discussion towards the next question, "Can you heed your own advice? If not, what stops you taking your own advice?"

A number of reasons are commonly given for not being able to take the advice that would be given to a friend. First, the patient states she is not able to think of it at the time. Second, she feels she has too much emotion and so cannot think. Third, she does not care what happens. Finally, everything happens so quickly that it is like a reflex. The clinician asks the patients to discuss in more detail the reasons for not being able to follow best advice and identifies the adverse consequences of different actions.

◆ Finding a solution.

> The clinician ends the task by asking the patients now to focus on different responses.

- What happens if I make this response? How does the outcome differ if I make an alternative response? Can I practice that response? Do I need to consider other problems, such as how I manage my feelings?

Sensitivity and interpersonal problems

Patients with BPD show marked sensitivity to others and may even have brief paranoid episodes. These are short-lived, triggered by environmental or interpersonal situations, and tend to respond rapidly to a change in circumstance (Gunderson & Lyons-Ruth, 2008). It is for this reason that we discuss sensitivity to others when discussing relationships. Patients with BPD are often strongly affiliative, seeking out relationships despite past negative relationship experiences.

When training clinicians in SCM we instruct them to focus carefully on interactions between patient and clinician and between group members in the problem-solving/advocacy group. Of particular note for people with BPD is their understanding of what others intend when the other person says or does something. All of us use two levels of information to decide this. First, we note external signals such as body movement, tone of voice, posture, and other visible or audible components of expression. Second, we consider the person's thoughts and feelings and our knowledge of their experiences. This internal–external distinction is particularly relevant in helping us to understand the paradoxical situation that some patients appear impaired in their capacity to understand what others mean or intend and may misinterpret things and yet are simultaneously highly sensitive and accurately pick up someone else's emotional state. They are showing hypersensitivity to people based primarily on external signals, observations of facial expression or lack of it or bodily posture. Patients with BPD find it very difficult to understand the intentions of others, an internally-based task (e.g., (King-Casas et al., 2008), even though they are often hypersensitive to some facial emotion expressions, an externally-based task (Lynch, et al., 2006; Domes et al., 2008; Domes, Schulze, & Herpertz, 2009). As we have mentioned, people with BPD tend to consider neutral facial expressions as indicating higher levels of threat than the general population does. By contrast, patients with antisocial personality disorder may lack the ability to read fearful emotions from facial expressions (an externally-based task) (Marsh & Blair, 2008), but they are often experts in reading the inner states of others, using this information and ability to achieve their interpersonal goals (Bateman & Fonagy, 2008a).

> The clinician outlines the internal and external cues that we use to understand others.

It is in this context that the clinician needs to work with patients to help them reflect on the immediacy and flexibility or rigidity of their conclusions about the intent of others.

> The clinician asks the group to give examples of when they have misunderstood the motive of someone close to them or when they have relied mostly on external cues.

The group then discuss what signals they are using to inform their interpretation of events and the intent of the other person. Many patients with BPD decide on someone's intent by their actions—"Peter didn't want to see me, otherwise why would he have forgotten about our meeting?" This should be questioned in the group.

> Are there other reasons why Peter could have forgotten about the meeting?

Using other examples, did the patients use mostly external cues or were they trying to find out what was going on in the mind of the other person and, if so, how did they do this? A list of ways of reconciling external indicators with internal states of the other to become more accurate about intent and meaning is generated. The following are some of the methods used in everyday life:

- Ask questions—"Why are you folding your arms?", "Why do you look at me like that?", "What are you thinking?"
- State a tentative conclusion and ask for confirmation—"I suppose that you feel that . . . . Is that what you do feel/think at the moment or are you feeling/thinking something else?"
- Explain how when someone says something or looks at you in a particular way that this results in certain emotions in oneself—"When you say that, I feel . . . Is that what you mean me to feel?"
- Explain your point of view—if it is not in line with what the other person means ask them to correct you.
- Consider the context of the interaction.

Self-harm

Information for the clinician

The following section may be photocopied and given to patients and so is provided on a separate page.

What is self-harm?

Self-harm is when someone intentionally hurts or harms themselves in a manner that results in damage to body tissue. People do this in many different ways, including:

+ taking too many tablets
+ cutting themselves
+ burning their body
+ banging their heads
+ throwing their body against something
+ punching themselves
+ sticking things in their body
+ swallowing objects.

Self-harm may be planned in advance or done suddenly with little thought, usually when emotions are strong. Some people might self-harm only once or twice but for others it can become a regular occurrence and feel like an addiction.

A broader definition of self-harm may include something we all do to a greater or lesser extent and some behavior can be less obvious as a form of self-harm simply because it seems socially acceptable to some peer groups. But it is often no less serious. For example, people can behave in ways that suggest they don't care whether they live or die. They may take drugs recklessly, frequently have sex with strangers or become "bug" chasers, gambling with being infected with sexually transmitted disease, or binge drink. Some people may restrict their eating as a way of self-harm.

Other names have been used to describe acts of self-harm without the intention to die and you may read the phrase "deliberate self-harm" (DSH) or the terms "parasuicide" and "attempted suicide". Sometimes the term "deliberate self-harm" can be used pejoratively or in a minimizing manner, which is unfortunate as self-harm describes an action that is a response to excruciatingly painful mental problems and is associated with a 30-fold increased rate of future suicide—indicator of the severity and importance of the problem. Whilst self-harm may be associated with suicidal intent or action, most self-harm in people with BPD is not an attempt at suicide and so the terms "parasuicide" and "attempted suicide" can be misleading where there is no suicidal intent. Do remember also that some people self-harm to keep away serious suicidal thoughts and that the patient's and clinician's view of suicidal intent might differ. Finally, the differentiation between self-harm and suicide attempts is not easily made and it is important to remember that suicide remains second only to accidental death as the leading cause of mortality in young men across the world, even though suicide rates for young men have fallen in some high-income and middle-income countries over the last decade. High-lethality methods of suicide are preferred by young men: hanging and firearms in high-income countries, pesticide poisoning in the Indian subcontinent, and charcoal-burning in east Asia (Pitman, Krysinska, Osborn, & King, 2012).

Who self-harms?

Recent research suggests that about 10% of young people self-harm (Hawton, Saunders, & O'Connor, 2012) but it can occur in any age group. Some self-harm may be culturally normative and not indicative of any problems (e.g., some adolescent subcultures). It is more common in females than males, although this might be more apparent than real, with men self-harming in different ways or explaining things away as accidents. Some groups, such as young South Asian women in the UK, seem to be more likely to self-harm than others, perhaps because of intercultural stresses. Sometimes groups of young people self-harm together and having a friend who self-harms may increase the chance of doing it as well. People who self-harm in ways that are not culturally normative are more likely to have experienced physical or sexual abuse during childhood, although many do not have such histories.

Research in hospital samples probably underestimates how common self-harm is, with surveys finding higher rates in communities and schools than in hospitals. Some forms of self-harm, such as cutting, may be more secret and so present to services less. In a recent study of over 4000 adults presenting with self-harm to hospital, overdose accounted for nearly 80% of episodes and cutting for only 15% but the situation is probably reversed in the community.

Many people self-harm just once or a few times; on the other hand once someone has started a pattern of self-harm they tend to self-harm again quite quickly and around 30% of people repeat self-harm over the following year.

Why do people self-harm?

We don't know precisely why people self-harm, but we do know that for many it alleviates distress in the short term. There is no single cause and there are very individual reasons as to why people self-harm. We do know that self-harm is linked with emotional distress and that people are struggling with difficulties for a period of time before they self-harm. There are often problems in relationships with partners, friends, and family, particularly in young people, who report feeling "not heard," hopeless, isolated, out of control and powerless. Unaddressed problems at school, such as bullying, or difficulties adjusting to college and university may also contribute. Self-harm can rapidly bring back a feeling of being in control, reduce tension, and relieve unbearable anguish and so easily becomes a "quick fix" for inner turmoil.

People are more likely to self-harm if they become depressed or abuse alcohol or drugs to any great extent.

Sometimes people appear to self-harm to show someone else how distressed they are or to get back at them but this is less common than people think. The majority of people suffer self-harm in silence.

The risk of a patient killing themselves increases if they are engaging in self-harm behaviors and so everyone who self-harms should be taken seriously and the events discussed in individual and group psychotherapy. Self-harm represents a problem in itself and so needs special consideration irrespective of any other areas of difficulty.

What can the patient do to help herself to reduce self-harm?

We know that urges to self-harm go down after a period of time and if the patient can cope with the immediate feelings without self-harming it will become easier over the next few hours. During this critical time the patient can try to take their mind off self-harm and specifically do something nice for themselves. Here are some suggestions for you to talk to the patient about:

- Talk to someone—if you are on your own perhaps phone a friend or if the person you are with is resulting in an increase in your distress then leave the situation for a time.
- Invoke your very own crisis plan.
- Distract yourself by going out, singing or listening to music, or by doing any activity that interests you.
- Relax and focus your mind on something pleasant—your very own personal comforting place.
- Find alternative outlets for the strong feelings, such as medically safe vigorous exercise, squeezing ice cubes (which you can make with red juice to mimic blood if the sight of blood is important) or even writing a strong letter to your psychiatrist/therapist expressing your feelings if relevant.
- Focus on positives if you can.
- Write a diary explaining to someone else what is going on.
- Contact self-harm helplines.
- Contact someone with whom you have a pre-arrangement about help.
- Write to yourself about the urge to self-harm or represent the urge in other ways by making collages or drawings.
- Make a tape of yourself, outlining good things about yourself and the reasons why you don't want to self-harm. Alternatively, ask a close person to do this for you and to remind you in the tape of your desirable characteristics.

When the urge is not so strong and the patient feels safe she should reflect in more detail on what happened and identify useful responses. These should be brought back to the group discussion.

What if the patient doesn't want to stop self-harming?

If the patient really decides that they don't want to stop self-harming it is best to help them to minimize the damage to their body by reducing the frequency and severity if they can. But better still is to keep reviewing why the patient is self-harming and revisiting their decision not to stop. In the end self-harm can be very damaging physically and psychologically, and people do better by stopping. Because self-harm is effective in decreasing distress, self-harm actions prevent the patient focusing on exploring alternative solutions to their problems, including ways of effectively tending to distressing emotions.

There are a number of questions the patient can ask themselves to see if they are ready to stop. Give them these questions and if they answer half of them 'yes' they should be encouraged to try to stop.

- Are there at least two people who are willing to help me stop?
- Is there a support network of friends that know about my self-harm and that I can go to if I get desperate?
- Have I found at least two alternative safe ways to reduce the feelings that lead me to self-harm?
- Am I able to tell myself and to believe it that I want to stop hurting myself?
- Can I tell myself that I *will* tolerate feelings of frustration, desperation, fear, and other distress?
- If necessary is there a professional who will also give me support and help in a crisis?
- Am I willing to minimize the harm?

Don't:

- speak out impulsively without reflection if you have strong emotions as this may result in the patient feeling worse
- expect them to stop overnight—stopping is difficult and takes time and effort
- make them promise not to do it again or make your offer of treatment contingent on an agreement for stopping
- make yourself responsible for the self-harm or become the person who is supposed to stop them.

Approach to self-harm in individual and group discussion

There is no single intervention for self-harm and most studies have suggested that treatment is difficult. Talking about the problem can help you clarify the areas of difficulty. Many episodes of self-harm are a result of a crisis in a close relationship. If this is the case discuss the relationship to see if this is leading to self-harm.

It is best to develop a crisis plan (see section on crisis planning in Chapter 3) about the self-harm which might suggest that the patient contacts someone to help ride the urge to self-harm and to give time for the urge to self-harm to go down.

The commonest technique used by clinicians in the generalist psychiatric service is the chain analysis. This can be used in both the problem-solving group and individual sessions. The technique is described in further detail in Chapter 8.

Chain analysis consists of naming elements in a chain of events and linking them together so an apparently isolated event is placed within a context. This is a powerful method of capturing the events leading up to self-harm or to other actions so it is a technique that is useful throughout treatment whenever a patient talks about "what she did or what happened."

Often the patient will say that they just "felt bad" and found themselves cutting, overdosing or risk-taking with no obvious context. Working through the incidents of the preceding period—minutes, hours or days—the therapist can identify salient events. The salience can be highlighted and then used as a focus for problem-solving work later. Once salient points or patterns are identified, they are noted on a piece of paper. Over time, a map of the pattern of the chain of events often emerges.

Chapter 5

Structured clinical management: team strategies

Summary

A rationale for teamwork is provided and suggestions are given about how to work together in a team when treating people with BPD.

Clinicians working in a team treating people with BPD need to agree to a common language and we recommend a focus on mentalizing as a basis for good teamwork. This provides structure without stricture and encourages a plurality of intervention.

Mentalizing refers to our ability to attend to mental states in ourselves and others, and is at the heart of team work. Mentalizing teams show:

- united mind with a commonality of purpose
- respect for themselves and others
- the ability to develop and adhere to coherent clinical plans
- good team morale
- effective leadership.

Team meetings can be organized around:

- identifying and marking the task
- stating the focus for discussion
- discussing the team's perspectives on the focus
- returning to task to link the discussion with the focus
- defining practical and clinical action.

One theme running through this book has been our emphasis on the need for clinicians to structure, coordinate, and integrate service provision for people with BPD. This is, in part, why the term "structured clinical management" was used in contrast to general psychiatric management. All specialist treatments for BPD, whatever theory underpins them, pay particular attention to coordination between the different clinicians involved. To put this into practice all clinicians must actively participate in teamwork; because of its importance we have devoted this chapter to the topic.

Rationale for teams

All of the evidence-based treatments for BPD emphasize teamwork in some form or another as an essential part of treatment. The emphasis ranges from teams delivering an overall treatment program (dialectical behavior therapy and mentalization-based therapy, for example) to individual therapists having regular supervision or consultation (transference-focused psychotherapy and schema-focused therapy, for example).

Linehan originally included team meetings in her research treatment protocol to maximize adherence to the model at that time and not as part of the treatment, but rapidly realized that the team was an essential part of the treatment going way beyond just ensuring what was considered adherence at the time. Teamwork is now an essential part of DBT adherence. The functioning of the team delivering DBT now holds equal place as one of the four essential components of standard DBT.

Despite this early recognition of the importance of a team, there remains no empirical evidence as far as we know demonstrating the importance of the team in the treatment of BPD and there is little robust evidence for positive effects of teamwork in outcomes of other disorders (Franx, Kroon, & Grimshaw, 2008). No dismantling studies have been done to identify the effect of teamwork. Evidence for the importance of teamwork in the treatment of BPD comes from the experience of organizing evidence-based treatments and delivering them effectively and from expert consensus that includes the views of both patients and clinicians.

Experts are agreed that the emotional difficulties engendered in clinicians during the treatment of people with BPD, the complexity of the relational processes, and concerns about risk all indicate that team support for the clinician is necessary. Clinicians need support to remain in the therapeutic relationship, to keep out of untherapeutic interactions, to be able to think about their work, and to deliver interventions sensitively and effectively. The team becomes the context in which a group of professionals deliver treatment. This is not to suggest that the individual clinician cannot treat people for BPD, but instead that a clinician working alone should use consultation with another clinician to support their work when treating high-risk patients with BPD. Gutheil (1989) and others (Norris, Gutheil, & Strasburger, 2003) identified a number of patient factors, such as "neediness and/or dependency, boundary confusion, previous sexual abuse, and entitlement," which placed a patient at risk of boundary violations from clinicians. Equally, if not more important, are factors in the clinician who, when working alone or unsupervised, may unwittingly become embroiled in boundary problems. The clinician's own life crises, a tendency to idealize a "special" patient or an inability to define personal and professional limits clearly, and denial about the possibility of boundary problems, all contribute. The clinician needs to be able to recognize his or her own capacities and ensure that these are not extended to breaking point—what can I manage and what am I comfortable with, for example, when considering between-session crisis contact.

A trainee working with a patient with BPD to support her in her transition from hospital to home following an admission to reduce her suicidal risk agreed to six sessions in his outpatient clinic. During the fifth session the patient requested some additional sessions because she had been doing well but thought that some further work would be extremely helpful. She flattered the trainee in terms of his skills and he readily agreed to more sessions. A few months later he realized that he had become very interested in the patient's life and the patient reported finding the sessions beneficial. He extended the session from 30 minutes, the normal length of an outpatient clinic appointment, to 50 minutes, the normal length of a psychotherapy session, and moved the appointment to the end of the clinic. At a later session the patient reported feeling suicidal so the trainee gave extra time. At the end of the session she told him that he had saved her life and she gave him a hug as she left, saying that their relationship had become so special to her that she thought about him constantly—in short she was in love with him. The trainee panicked and asked for supervision from a senior colleague.

A team can protect the clinician from a potential slippery slope which, if unchecked, can culminate in boundary violations (Gutheil, 1989). In the example above, extending the number of sessions was the first indicator of a potential boundary crossing and this was rapidly followed by extending the length of sessions. A team would have been alert to these "clinically driven" decisions and questioned them carefully. Clinicians working in a team are required to report their work on a regular basis. The patient will often see other members of the team, in a crisis for example, who can pick up early warning signs of problems. But it is probably the support role of the team that is most important and helps the clinician remain focused on treatment and balanced in the relationship with the patient, avoiding becoming overly close or excessively distant.

Coordination

People with BPD, because of their numerous problems, attract multiple mental health professionals from different training backgrounds—nurses, psychologists, psychiatrists, social care workers, probation officers, housing support officers to name but a few—all of whom have different theoretical perspectives, diverse support structures, and independent management and governance pathways, making general psychiatric management problematic. Under these conditions it is not surprising that contradictory advice is often given to patients. It is challenging to ensure that the interventions delivered by such a disparate group of clinicians correspond and, in doing so, coalesce into a coherent whole. This is the reason why we recommend a coordinated and functioning team for the structured clinical management of people with BPD. The primary role of the team is to deliver effective care for people with BPD in the context of having access to only limited additional training beyond levels acquired during generic trainings. And yet this team will have to ensure that integration of a wider network is well managed. This will involve family and friends, who are of primary importance in any treatment process and we discuss this separately in Chapter 7.

This type of uncoordinated advice is harmful to people with BPD. All clinicians working with patients with BPD need to be aware that they are better to say to a patient that they will discuss the different options with others involved in treatment first and then again with the patient once this has been done. This allows a considered response with a tangible rationale to be given. Inevitably this process is easier if a team is working together to deliver care. Eventually the whole team promote the patient, integrating their own treatment rather than acting on their behalf and this includes encouraging them to approach some of the people outside the core treatment team.

A common language for teams

SCM of people with BPD requires effective teamwork. In Chapter 2 we outlined some of the characteristics of clinicians that are likely to lead to good team function. All clinicians should have chosen to work with people with BPD, be enthusiastic about the work, optimistic about outcomes, compassionate, and willing to organize around a shared understanding of the disorder. We consider mentalizing a suitable bedrock on which to build effective teamwork simply because using mentalizing brings a specific attitude to clinicians and can act as a framework or "glue" that joins together teams, their work, and their interventions without insisting individual clinicians give up their own way of working. The plurality and permissiveness of the mentalizing frame provides structure without unnecessary stricture. General mental health clinicians can maintain their current practice without feeling deskilled and retain a level of comfort in treating people with BPD that can be lost if they feel that they have to radically change their way of working.

Mentalizing

Mentalizing lies at the very core of our humanity—it refers to our ability to attend to mental states in ourselves and in others as we attempt to understand our own actions and those of others on the basis of intentional mental states

(Bateman & Fonagy, 2012). This fundamental process lies at the heart of team-work and is an integrative mechanism underpinning not only the generic and specific strategies of SCM discussed in earlier chapters but also the team inter-action. Mentalizing as an essential process can often be signed up to by a wide network of professionals who are organized around a person with BPD. All interactions with the patient, whether stemming from a team member or from the wider network, are directed towards stimulating and sustaining mentaliza-tion in the patient. Mentalizing serves as a "common currency" or language throughout the team (Bateman & Fonagy, 2012). Specifically, team members should see their responsibility as being not only to increase or sustain mentaliz-ing in their patients, but also in themselves and their professional colleagues.

Mentalizing techniques focus practitioner–patient interaction on the sub-jective and phenomenological mental experience of the patient. This will improve the patient experience of treatment. There is a need for any prac-titioner to see the world from the patient's perspective. Whenever the focus on the patient's internal mental process is dominant there is intrinsic value because of the powerful commitment to the patient's subjectivity but, in addi-tion, working to enhance a patient's mentalizing capacity will potentially make general approaches more effective. A team need to commit to trying to under-stand the subjective experience of the patient and to find the reality within it whilst simultaneously pledging to engage in a parallel process themselves by continuously undertaking a process of self-observation. The overall aim is to develop a team with a united mind.

United mind

A commonality of purpose in a team and coherent responses to a wide range of clinical situations can only come about if a team function with one mind whilst retaining their own individuality. To do so, a team need to follow some basic principles. First, respect of each other has to be apparent and worked on rather than assumed. Second, the team need constantly to define and redefine their aims with each patient; these aims have to be consistent with the overall aims of the treatment process. Third, the team must emphasize communica-tion between each other. All members hold equal responsibility for ensuring information, ideas, and plans are shared appropriately. Finally, leadership and support structures need agreement. All members have to be committed to working within them—mavericks are welcome but loose cannons will destroy a team which may never recover. The identified team lead does not have to be the permanent lead of team discussions. Well-functioning teams show flexible processes rather than strict hierarchical structures and the lead of a discussion may be someone identified at the beginning of a team meeting or be identified on a rotational basis, for example.

Respect

Respect means each team member gives appropriate regard to others team members' feelings, opinions, and experience. All clinicians are aware that people with BPD can evoke contradictory feelings in an individual and this inevitably becomes apparent between team members. One team member may be enraged with a patient whilst another feels highly protective; patients may engage one member of the team by outlining—perhaps exaggerating—the shortcomings of another member of the team. For the unwary, this can have a seductive quality as criticism of a "rival" promises the potential of clinical "riches" in becoming special to a patient. Sometimes the criticisms of a colleague, reported in a clinical session, are highly accurate and may even hit sensitive differences between members of the team. Of course this cuts both ways and the same patient may be reversing the criticisms when seeing another team member. An explicit and collective refusal to be drawn into these subtly subversive conversations improves the chances of effective team functioning. Integrating the views of the patient and the reciprocal reactions of the clinicians to the patient perspective is a key function of the team. Valuing another view, however different from your own, maintains the respect required to facilitate an integrated view of a patient's psychological function.

Clinical planning

Successful planning needs organizational support for team meetings and an explicit statement to all team members about the emphasis in practice on taking into account different clinical perspectives. The team organize themselves around the problems of the patient and begin a process of integrating different ideas and clinical suggestions. Often this can be done with the patient who, detached from the emotional intensity of team interactions, may be able to benefit from observing others discuss alternative ideas about help which gradually coalesce into a practical and meaningful plan to which everyone can commit.

One patient informed a member of the team that she brought a knife to sessions in her bag as she felt unsafe on the streets and felt more secure in therapy sessions with the knife in her bag. The clinician was concerned not only because carrying an offensive weapon is illegal but also for her own safety in the session. It was a concern to the team for exactly the same reasons and worries were expressed that the clinician would not be able to focus on the patient's treatment whilst she was so concerned that the patient was carrying a knife. The team were uncertain what to do, so organized a meeting of the whole team with the patient to discuss the matter. An array of opinions was expressed, ranging from discharging the patient unless she promised not to carry knives to sessions to more protective comments about the patient's anxieties. The process of discussion enabled the patient to realize that the states of mind she was evoking in the team were untenable for continuing treatment and she agreed never to bring weapons to sessions. The process of discussion allowed all participants to believe her statement was an accurate reflection of change rather than a mere glib and superficial statement with no basis in future reality.

Supporting the team

Team morale

People working with patients with personality disorder can easily become demoralized for a number of reasons and team support is essential. First, people with BPD are emotionally challenging to work with, at times picking on staff members, finding their weak spots, threatening them, challenging their therapeutic zeal, evoking negative emotions (including frustration), countertransference feelings, and becoming dismissive of their work. Conversely, patients may make a team member feel special, important, powerful, and even as someone essential to their survival. It is understandable that these extreme patterns in therapeutic relationships emerge in treatment, given the emotional and interpersonal nature of BPD, but it is the response of the clinician that holds the key to managing the problem. Clinicians have a tendency to react by trying to achieve more and more, placing unrealistic demands on themselves and even trying, in the face of feelings of incompetence, to be seen as a "good" clinician. These responses are balanced by team discussion and brought back into perspective so that the clinician does not feel inadequate in the face of stressful demands and refrains from engaging in short-term solutions (for example gaining favor by acquiescing to demands for admission to hospital for suicidality), which harms development of personal strategies useful for the long term. Second, change in personality disorder is slow and, at times, clinicians and patients have to recognize that considerable work is repeated without obvious benefit; working on the same problem within different contexts is commonplace and necessary. Whilst repetition might seem disheartening at first, and it is not uncommon to hear statements from clinicians such as "we've been here before," "this is the same old pattern," it is also a chance to revisit the problem when it is "hot," allowing another opportunity for change and development. Again, it is the team that help the clinician not react with frustration. Third, splits within the team commonly manifest themselves as disagreements which may become polarized, making it hard for individuals not to blame each other for management or treatment difficulties. Fourth, the fluctuating nature of the problems of the person with BPD and the intermittent crises can lead to an onerous workload and constant anxiety about risk. Finally, a suicide of a patient not only has a profound effect on the individual who was treating the patient but also on the whole team, who might blame themselves, might feel that they will be blamed by others, and will have to face a psychological autopsy in which all aspects of the treatment of the patient is reviewed. The effect that all these factors have on the individual and team is determined in part by the function of the team itself. A team working cohesively looks after its members, protects them, helps them understand what is happening or has happened, gives a member a rest when necessary, allows time for further training, and ensures that any one individual is not overburdened with high-risk patients.

Leadership

A team needs constant attention to maintain smooth functioning and consideration should be given to how it is structured. Leadership is needed at different levels. Within the team it should come from the most experienced and senior professional whose task is to preserve the structure of the treatment program, support staff, supervise on an everyday basis, and treat the more problematic patients. Leadership of the service rests in the person who is best placed to offer expert supervision, who can negotiate within the system, and who has the respect of all staff. Leadership is given rather than taken or assumed because of professional identity. The qualities of a good leader are not specific to any one professional group and are related more to some of the personal qualities identified earlier that are important in the treatment of people with BPD.

Clear leadership is necessary to ensure the agreed protocols are implemented between groups throughout the system. Leadership requires a willingness on the part of team members to assign the responsibility of leadership to a member of the team as well as that member being willing to undertake the leadership role. Underlying rivalries within a team will inevitably bring with them inconsistency as members of the team attempt to develop greater influence. The natural tendency to want to make an individual contribution has to become subdominant to the team itself. In order to achieve this, development of an iterative process is necessary in which the team move towards a consensus that is then held by the team itself. New members of the team can then be educated by the team in the team perspective.

Sustaining team enthusiasm and morale is primarily through an admixture of serious work with supervision, provision of time for private learning, and the development of a space to laugh and cry together. The latter is rarely discussed openly but there is no doubt that a team that can laugh together and be sad with each other about their professional trials and tribulations as well as some of their personal concerns when appropriate will function supportively and effectively. The humanity of a team will create a secure atmosphere within the treatment milieu, allowing disagreement between therapists to take place in safety, for example during a group therapy session, and the facilitation of a questioning culture.

In an advocacy group session focusing on managing interactions with social services, one of the therapists made a statement in the group that was followed by silence. The other therapist sensed that the patients had not understood what was said and in fact he had not done so himself. He said to the therapist "I didn't understand a word of that, do you think you could try again to explain what you were trying to say." The therapist laughed and said "I wasn't sure that I understood it either so maybe it is a good idea to start again." This not only allowed the patients to realize that staff could be muddled or at least could obfuscate things but also demonstrated that it was possible to question things constructively and to stimulate further thought rather than to dismiss or ignore what was said.

Team meetings

Many teams follow an agreed protocol in clinical meetings and we outline here some suggestions for this based on work with young people with emerging personality disorder (Bevington, in press). First, it is important that the clinicians who want to discuss a clinical problem make it known at the beginning of the meeting. It is surprising how often people bring up some complex clinical problem just before a meeting finishes! Second, the clinician identifies or "marks" the task. Third, she states her case. Fourth, there is general discussion which enables all team members involved in the treatment of the patient to offer their perspective. Team members not involved "mentalize the discussion" by ensuring that all views are respected and that the emotional support the clinician needs is addressed. Finally the team return to task to answer the initial questions posed by the clinician.

Identifying and marking the task

Once team members have expressed a wish to discuss a clinical problem and the order of discussion has been agreed the team must help the clinician explicitly identify the problem and what she wants out of the discussion. Too often clinicians and teams revert to story-telling. Whilst this has merits, particularly in helping clinicians ventilate their feelings and to feel validated, it is unlikely to lead to practical and effective ongoing treatment planning. This is why marking the task is necessary and is the responsibility of the presenting clinician. In the earlier example, the clinician identified her concerns about the patient carrying a knife and marked the task as being about how she managed this practically and how she processed her fearfulness in the session. Additional examples of marking a task are:

> *I would like to discuss the level of risk of this patient and decide on how to address it.*
> *I would value how to increase this patient's level of motivation for treatment and discuss what I can do or even do less of to improve attendance.*
> *I am anxious before seeing this patient. During the session I am very careful about what I say. I feel reticent about challenging her and I would like to think more about that.*

Stating the case

The clinician then briefly presents the clinical problem without interruption. The veto on interruption is important because too many diversions from the task will prevent effective presentation of the problem as the clinician experiences it. Equally, the clinician has to ensure that the presentation of the problem does not drift into story-telling but focuses on the identified task.

Discussion and mentalizing the process

Once the clinician has completed their presentation, the meeting is open to the team for comments and perspectives. Importantly, any team member who is not involved in the care of the patient acts as the guardian of the mentalizing process of the discussion, listening carefully for "absolutes" and extreme views (for example "she is just … ", "clearly he is . …) and quickly identifying them. Teams can easily and yet imperceptibly fall into a group process that demonizes patients with BPD, seeing the problems as the fault of the patient when in fact it is a problem within the team or the treatment plan. Organizing a team discussion so that dispassionate members of the team act as sentinels of the process is necessary to prevent this.

Return to task

The chair of the meeting takes charge of returning the team to task. Often this is best done by summarizing much of the discussion and linking it to the problem identified initially. An effort is required at this point to define clear practical actions and it is helpful to remember the START criteria around any planned task. The five aspects of START are Space (who?), Time (when?), Authority (who has authority?), Responsibility (who has responsibility?), and Task (what actions need to be done?).

Supervision

It is impossible to maintain team morale and to deliver effective treatment without supervision. It is all too easy for treatment to become chaotic, for clinicians to develop extreme or idiosyncratic views, individual members to feel victimized, patients to be turned into scapegoats, and mistakes made involving boundary transgressions. Supervision reduces the likelihood of these events and is best organized on a group and individual basis as an intrinsic part of any program for BPD.

Supervision needs to be considered in terms of the team itself. Formal supervision to the team about their clinical work is often provided by the leader of the service, which brings with it the danger of a closed system outside the scrutiny of others. To prevent the development of self-serving attitudes, the insidious formation of unquestioned beliefs, and the creation of a "corporate delusion," each team member may be offered individual supervision outside the treatment program with a senior clinician from a different but allied part of the mental health service. It is important that clinicians feel secure to discuss their own views, the problems they are having with a patient, and the difficulties they may be having with their own feelings about the patient or with implementing treatment. It also gives a chance to explain what they did, why they did it, what happens in sessions, and for their therapy to be questioned by an expert clinician, perhaps with an alternative perspective. Findings from the individual supervisions are brought together and considered within the framework of the supervision run by the service lead.

Supervision has a number of overlapping aims. First, it is a method to ensure that clinicians keep to a treatment plan and apply interventions appropriately, but it is important that therapists do not feel overscrutinized and criticized when they inevitably deviate. Divergence is inevitable because it is easy for a therapist to become drawn into nontherapeutic interventions. Second, it is a place in which the therapist should feel free to discuss the major evolving themes along with his responses to the patient. Third, supervision needs to support and to challenge. Simply giving encouragement does not increase skill and may even perpetuate bad habits, so a secure atmosphere in which both the supervisor and supervisee can question each other is necessary. Fourth, the supervision can be used to understand the patient/clinician relationship. The relationship that the therapist makes in supervision may, in part, reflect the underlying problem in treatment itself.

One supervisee became very challenging in supervision, expressing concern that nothing that the supervisor said seemed to help him orientate his mind to tackle the next contact with the patient. At first the supervisor tried to make more and more suggestions until he realized that this may be exactly what was happening in therapy—the clinician was giving more and more support to the patient but felt that it was increasingly ineffective. This parallel process identified in individual supervision was then used to discuss the problem in the team meeting.

How often supervision occurs will be dependent on the level of training and experience but all clinicians, even the most experienced and best trained, should have individual supervision and/or participate in group peer–peer supervision. New staff will need more support and guidance.

Chapter 6

Structured clinical management: inpatient treatment and prescribing

Summary

Acute inpatient treatment is not recommended as a treatment of choice for people with BPD but it may be necessary at times.

Indicators for acute hospital admission may include:

◆ acute suicide risk

◆ imminent danger of extremely risky behavior

◆ onset of severe depression and other comorbidity

◆ review and rationalization of medication

◆ feelings in the clinician and rupture of the therapeutic relationship.

Acute suicide risk needs to be differentiated from chronic risk.

Warning signs that a long-term risk is becoming more acute should be incorporated into a crisis plan and identified early in treatment.

Possible indicators of acute risk include:

◆ direct suicide statements

◆ deteriorating major depression

◆ deteriorating substance abuse

◆ negative life events

◆ lowering of family/peer support

◆ increasing symptoms

◆ sudden detachment with a breakdown in therapeutic alliance

◆ feelings in the clinician.

The aims of hospital admission are to:

◆ decrease risk to a level manageable in the community

◆ reduce or disrupt a cycle of risky behavior

- treat a severe co-occurring disorder
- manage severe alcohol and/or substance abuse
- review and stabilize medication
- manage the feelings of the clinician.

Prescribing medication to people with BPD is associated with numerous problems.

Reasons for prescribing are often unclear and may be determined as much by the problems experienced by the clinician as those faced by the patient.

Medication should be considered in the context of a long-term treatment plan and caution taken when prescribing when a patient is in a crisis.

Prescribers need to beware of prescribing due to patient demand or in response to pleas from other mental health professionals.

Prescribing may need to be informed by the clinician's underlying feelings, for example a strong wish to signify care in the context of complaints that not enough is being done.

Prescribing should be done within carefully negotiated and agreed parameters.

Inpatient treatment

One of the primary aims of SCM is to reduce unnecessary hospital admissions for patients with BPD. With this aim, treatment is organized to manage crises without resorting to admission whenever possible. Crisis plans are developed, vulnerability factors of the patient are identified to use as an early warning system, and ways of managing emotional distress are developed. Yet, at times, admission to hospital may become necessary. We consider here the role of hospital admission. But first a brief caution is necessary.

Iatrogenesis

There are many reasons to avoid hospital admission. Expert consensus, not always reliable but in this case matching the best available evidence, suggests that acute inpatient care is often suboptimal for the treatment of people with BPD. At best it is neutral for the patient's long-term development; at worst it is damaging. Nonetheless it can, of course, also be life-saving in the short term when used judiciously.

Interestingly, whilst some studies of residential therapy have been favorable (see (Lees, Manning, & Rawlings (1999) for review), other studies suggest that long-term residential treatment in a specialist treatment centre may also fail to generate positive long-term benefits, suggesting that the problem may not be simply the lack of skills of staff on an acute ward who may know little about BPD. A study carried out by the Cassel Hospital/UCL research group has shown that personality disorder patients exposed to a step-down program comprising a short/medium inpatient stay in a therapeutic community setting followed by long-term outpatient treatment improve on a number of indicators (global functioning, symptom severity, social adjustment, and recidivism). In contrast, long-term inpatient treatment (>6 months) yielded disappointing results, with a third of patients improving, a third not changing, and a third getting worse. Deliberate self-injury and readmission to hospital did not improve in the long-term inpatient cohort (Chiesa, Fonagy, & Holmes, 2006; Chiesa, Fonagy, Holmes, & Drahorad, 2004).

The same group also investigated the impact of deliberate self-injury and treatment program allocation as moderating factors for outcome at 2-year follow-up. They found a significant three-way interaction between deliberate self-harm, treatment model, and outcome at 24-month follow-up. This means that patients presenting with greater severity of psychopathology do better if treated in a less intense community-based setting than if they are treated in a more intensive long-term residential program (Chiesa, Sharp, & Fonagy, 2011). While severity was a negative predictor of outcome for inpatient treatment, that was not the case for the community-based program.

A recently published Dutch nonrandomized multicentre study of Cluster A, B and C, personality disorder patients treated in different settings, compared the effectiveness of long-term outpatient (more than 6 months), short-term day hospital (up to 6 months), long-term day hospital, short-term inpatient, and long-term inpatient psychotherapy in terms of psychiatric symptoms, psychosocial functioning, and quality of life. The data add further complexity to concerns about inpatient treatment for people with personality disorder. For Cluster C disorders, the results showed that patients in all treatment groups had improved on all outcomes 12 months after baseline. However, patients receiving short-term inpatient treatment showed somewhat more improvement than patients receiving other treatment modalities (Bartak et al., 2010). With regard to Cluster B patients, after controlling for pretreatment differences, the differences in outcome between outpatient, day hospital, and inpatient treatment were nonsignificant (Bartak, Andrea, Spreeuwenberg, Ziegler, et al., 2011). In Cluster A patients, day hospital and inpatient treatment were superior to outpatient treatment, but differences at baseline between the samples and the small sample size limit this latter conclusion (Bartak, Andrea, Spreeuwenberg, Thunnissen, et al., 2011).

A recent study at Kortenberg Hospital near Brussels showed significant improvement in symptom severity, interpersonal functioning, general functioning, and self-harm at 12 months after the initial evaluation, following an average 6-month inpatient stay in a psychotherapy program (Vermote et al., 2009). However, the lack of control group limits the strength of the findings. Because it is well known that people with BPD and other personality factors are not a homogeneous group, Vermote and colleagues identified two groups of patients in this study. While one group showed sustained improvement in symptoms during treatment and follow-up, no improvement was found in the second group of patients. The group who benefited were those who presented primarily with problems regarding autonomy and self-definition, while those who did not benefit were patients with difficulties of dependency and "neediness." Even at 5-year follow-up the identification of this subgroup of patients who did not respond as well as the other group of patients to inpatient treatment was apparent, suggesting that the ill-effects were long lasting.

It looks like there is a principle of less is more. This beneficial outcome of "less" may be explained by the compounding effect of patient and therapist working again and again on managing emotional crises within an interpersonal and everyday social context rather than avoiding them by hospital admission. The patient incrementally generates his own coping mechanisms and develops constructive ways of avoiding the crisis in the first place.

There is indicative evidence over time that inpatient treatment may be harmful to patients with BPD although the evidence that it leads to regression, widely reported by clinicians, is not matched by research (Gabbard et al., 2000). Early follow-up studies, when many patients were treated as inpatients, highlighted the inexorable nature of the "disease," talking of "burnt out" borderlines and hinting less at recovery than at a disease process which ran a long-term course (Stone, 1990). Therapeutic nihilism abounded in the literature, justified by the clinicians' impotence in the face of a patient's emotional pain, the often dramatic self-mutilation, and the degree of ambivalence in engaging in therapy.

More recent studies have contradicted this early view. The majority of BPD patients experience a substantial reduction in their symptoms far sooner than previously assumed, as we discussed in Chapter 1 (see section on prognosis in Chapter 1). It transpires that after 6 years, 75% of patients diagnosed with BPD severe enough to require hospitalization achieve remission by standardized diagnostic criteria (Zanarini, et al., 2006). At 16-year follow-up assessment more than 78% of patients continued to show remission (range 78–99%). However, recovery of good psychosocial function was less apparent, with

40–60% achieving and continuing reasonable social and vocational function along with symptomatic relief (Zanarini, et al., 2012). Nevertheless, this data along with a further study on the longitudinal course of BPD (Gunderson et al., 2011) with better than expected outcomes suggest that patients with BPD undergo remission—a concept that had previously been solely used in the context of Axis I pathology. About 50% remission rate has occurred by 4 years but the remission rate is steady (10–15% per year). This contrasts with the natural course of many Axis I disorders, such as affective disorder, where improvement may be somewhat more rapid but recurrences are common (Keller et al., 1992). What is the explanation for this change?

One possible conclusion is that some psychosocial treatments practiced currently, and perhaps even more commonly in the past, have impeded the patient's capacity to recover following the natural course of the disorder and prevented them harnessing advantageous changes in social circumstances (Fonagy & Bateman, 2006). In Michael Stone's (Stone, 1990) classic follow-up of patients treated nearly 40 years ago, 66% recovery rate was only achieved after 20 years (four times longer than reported in more recent studies). Has the nature of the disorder changed? Have treatments become that much more effective? Both seem unlikely explanations. The known efficacy of pharmacological agents, new and old, cannot account for this difference (Tyrer & Bateman, 2004); the evidence-based psychosocial treatments are not widely available. Could the apparent improvement in the course of the disorder be accounted for by harmful treatments being less frequently offered? If correct, this change is possibly more a consequence of the changing pattern of financially driven healthcare, particularly in the USA than recognition by clinicians of the possibility of iatrogenic deterioration and subsequent avoidance of damaging side-effects. This suggestion is speculative but it requires further consideration even though evidence from the recent longitudinal studies does not tell us whether interventions that were delivered were effective or inappropriate and nor is it possible to determine exactly when improvement occurred in the older retrospective follow-up studies.

Indicators for hospital admission

Despite all the concerns about admission of patients to specialist inpatient treatment centers and to acute inpatient units, there are times when the clinician will need to suggest hospital admission. These include:

+ acute suicide risk
+ imminent danger of extremely risky behavior
+ onset of severe depression and other comorbidity

+ review and rationalization of medication
+ feelings in the clinician and rupture of the therapeutic relationship.

Acute suicide risk

The clinician should beware of admitting patients simply because they state suicidal thoughts. Until explored and proven otherwise, such suicidal thoughts should be taken as part of the long-term risk (Paris, 2003, 2004; Paris & Zweig-Frank, 2001). Inpatient admission is ineffective in reducing long-term suicide risk but may be necessary to manage acute risk. Increased major depression, substance abuse, negative life events, and decreased family support are associated with acute risk.

Assessing acute risk in patients with BPD is difficult due to the background of persistent long-term risky behavior and the frequent statements made by patients with BPD about being suicidal. These factors may inoculate the clinician against the level of risk and as a result she becomes insensitive and misses subtle changes in the patient's state of mind. The crisis plan (see section on crisis planning in Chapter 3) developed with the patient at the beginning of treatment will have taken into account the acute and chronic suicide risk and identified factors which increase and decrease risk. The clinician needs to be alert to events that increase risk whilst constantly ensuring mechanisms for reducing risk are in place. Whilst the latter often take the form of identifying clear pathways for support and making sure they are still open, they also include maintaining a good therapeutic relationship in treatment. Fractures in the therapeutic relationship are likely to increase risk rapidly.

Detailed delineation of events preceding previous suicide attempts will alert the clinician to future indicators of increased risk. The presence of any of these factors may help differentiate between the background risk and an immediate increased risk, and should signal to the clinician that further exploration of suicidal feelings and thoughts is necessary. Mounting levels of distress and symptom severity both indicate that risk is increasing. But the converse also probably holds true—beware the patient who suddenly becomes detached having been attached, has few symptoms having complained of extensive symptoms, whose mood is flat having been manifestly angry and depressed. Look for nonattendance, often with nonsubstantial reasons given, after a period of regular attendance. Look for any major change in social circumstances. Be alert to changes in professional support, for example a social worker or housing support officer leaving their employment. Patients with BPD are sensitive to change and can easily feel abandoned. Finally, note an increase in contact with services, for example frequent phone calls and/or emails. The patient may experience a need to be in contact with the clinician but not recognize or communicate that this is a precursor of suicidality.

A number of interventions are open to the clinician once a change in risk has been detected or the patient has stated explicitly he is suicidal. First, the clinician should immediately explore the patient's emotions, ask when they started and what was the context, and undertake a chain analysis of events (see section on chain analysis in Chapter 8) to see if the impulse to act can be diverted onto a less destructive path. Second, techniques to reduce hyperarousal should be implemented if needed. Third, any vulnerability factors that add to the risk should be addressed. Patients paradoxically increase their vulnerability to making a suicide attempt by the behaviors they deploy in a desperate attempt to reduce their distress. They smoke cannabis, take a cocktail of drugs or drink excessive amounts of alcohol; they withdraw from social contacts and retreat from supportive relationships. Only once these areas have been explored, addressed, and the interventions are not reducing the risk should the clinician begin to consider hospital admission.

Risky behavior

Clinicians tend to worry about suicidal statements rather than other risk-taking behaviors for obvious reasons. Some risk-taking behavior may become engrained into a patient's way of life—uncontrolled drug misuse without addiction, multiple sexual partners with unprotected sex, gambling, binge drinking, restrictive eating—and, as such becomes the background to treatment. Just as chronic suicide risk inoculates the clinician against being alert to risk (Gunderson, 2008), the clinician can become immune to the peril of other behaviors, gradually and imperceptibly becoming insensitive to their danger to the patient's health or life. The clinician fails to ask about the behaviors on a regular basis. Look for escalation; always explore the activity and its precipitants, if necessary asking the patient about them each week. As soon as the clinician begins to dismiss, or becomes excessively urbane about, a patient's risk activity, discussion should take place urgently in the team.

Comorbidity

In Chapter 1 we mentioned the frequent co-occurrence of other psychiatric disorders in people with BPD. Affective disorders and anxiety disorders are perhaps the most common (see also section on co-occurring conditions in Chapter 1). Whenever they co-occur clinicians will be faced with an increasingly complicated treatment process and may take refuge in hospital admission as the comorbidity increases the patient's vulnerability and decreases their ability to manage the stressors of everyday life.

Affective disorders

The onset of depression in BPD and its persistence, despite medication and other available treatment, must be taken seriously as risk increases markedly. Lack of motivation, inertia, and hopelessness may all prevent patients using skills to manage impulses and emotional storms, thus increasing the danger to themselves. Some clinicians suggest that feelings of persistent sadness and guilt, and a mood lacking in reactivity to personal circumstances and external events in a patient with BPD suggest that depression has been superimposed on the symptoms of BPD. On the other hand, symptoms of anger, loneliness, and emptiness are more likely to be part of the BPD itself (Gunderson & Phillips, 1991; Gunderson, et al., 2004). The good news is that if a patient with both BPD and depression is being treated for BPD and sees improvement in those BPD symptoms, the symptoms of depression also seem to lift. However, this effect seems to be unidirectional and if treatment is focused solely on depression the symptoms of BPD do not seem to improve (Gunderson, et al., 2008, 2011).

The co-occurrence or overlap of bipolar disorder with BPD remains controversial (Gunderson et al., 2006) but for a clinician the combination is likely to increase her heart rate at times as she tries to identify what is the reactivity of the BPD and what is a more persistent change in mood. The lifetime rate of co-occurrence of bipolar and BPD is suggested to be around 27.6%. This seems high enough to suggest a significant relationship; this may not be the case. Analyses of co-occurrence rates from multiple studies show that the rate of BPD comorbidity in bipolar patients is not higher than for patients with other personality disorders. In a study by Gunderson and colleagues the rate of bipolar co-occurrence in the BPD group was modest compared to the rates found for other disorders (Gunderson, et al., 2006). For example, in BPD patients, the rates of co-occurrence for major depressive disorder, substance abuse, and post-traumatic stress disorder (PTSD) were all more than twice the rate found for bipolar I and bipolar II disorder. Finally, because rates of co-occurrence are always elevated in clinical samples, good epidemiological data on the co-occurrence rates of these two disorders in healthy populations are needed before a relationship can be inferred. Nevertheless the clinician may be advised to consider hospital admission for patients who show persistently elevated mood and a grandiose sense of self along with increasing irritability and bouts of anger, particularly if the symptoms cause major disruption to the therapeutic alliance.

Sensitivity reactions

Acute sensitivity reactions in a patient can endanger the continuation of treatment, particularly if they involve the treating clinicians and they become frankly paranoid. Whilst these are often short-lived in patients with BPD, their sudden onset and ferocity can surprise even the most experienced clinician. Occasionally, hospital admission is necessary to disrupt the process and to stabilize medication whilst the trigger for the reaction is investigated. But generally it is best to try to retrieve the clinician–patient relationship without immediate hospital admission. Importantly, the clinician needs to actively search for her own contribution to the sensitivity reaction and *not* initially see it as something the patient has either misinterpreted or imagined.

Drugs and alcohol

Comorbid substance abuse and alcohol addiction require the clinician to assess the need for additional services and to consider referral to specialist treatment facilities for "detox" or rehabilitation. SCM actively promotes the effective use of other services by the patient. A need for additional services is not a reason to discharge the patient from treatment for their personality disorder but a way of cementing the therapeutic alliance and supporting the patient in using services appropriately.

Clinicians also need to consider less addictive drug and alcohol misuse as "risky behaviors" and not accept them as an inevitable consequence of emotional stress. Many patients smoke cannabis or use "skunk," a concentrated form of cannabis, on a regular basis or drink alcohol excessively, stating that these substances help them manage their emotions better. Whilst this may have some validity in some people in the short term, such substance use interferes with treatment and may indicate that admission to an acute psychiatric ward is necessary if they spiral out of control and lead to other risk-taking behavior.

Other personality disorders

Suicidal behavior may also increase as result of the comorbidity of BPD with other personality disorders. One of concern, discussed by clinicians but receiving scant empirical attention, is narcissistic personality disorder. Strong narcissistic characteristics, such as a grandiose sense of self and a belief of indestructibility sometimes associated with excessive pride and contempt for others, often including the clinician, makes successful treatment challenging. Accepting help can be experienced by the person with narcissistic personality disorder as a submission which undermines self-sufficiency and the grandiose sense of self. In addition, treatment threatens exposing flaws in the self. Eventually death may be seen as better than dishonor, so beware the patient who manifests marked narcissistic features during treatment; they may not have been apparent at assessment even during a structured interview but may be revealed as part of a depressed mood or interpersonal stressor (Miller, Campbell, & Pilkonis, 2007). In a study of mentalization-based treatment for BPD, increasing comorbidity for personality disorders from different Clusters reduced responsiveness to treatment (Bateman & Fonagy, in press) and Kvarstein and Karterud (2012) found that Cluster C personality disorder predicted poorer outcomes in a large cohort of patients with mixed personality disorders.

Review of medication

We discuss the use of medication for BPD later in this chapter. Suffice to say here that the problems encountered with the use of medication in the treatment of BPD can necessitate admission to rationalize previously unsafe prescribing. Patients present to services on a cocktail of drugs, some of which may lead to serious withdrawal effects. Benzodiazepines, for example, are used more often than is appropriate and some patients become reliant on their anxiolytic effect. Safe reduction over time is necessary and although this can often be done as an outpatient, a short period of inpatient treatment might be necessary.

Rationalizing a patient's medication can also usually be done as an outpatient but, again, for the safety of the patient and their own reassurance, this might need hospital admission.

Feelings in the clinician

Naturally, clinicians tend to seek factors in the patient to inform them about the need for admission. Yet the experience of the clinician may also signal serious problems (Betan, Heim, Conklin, & Westen, 2005). Paris (2003) has suggested that there is an increase in risk for patients with BPD who come to an end of a series of failed treatments. The beginning of the end may start in the clinician before the patient. Giving up on the patient, considering them untreatable, wanting to refer them to someone else in the middle of their treatment program, and dreading treatment sessions may all indicate that there is a problem within the patient–therapist relationship, which in itself might increase the risk of the patient. The feelings of the clinician may become so powerful that a rupture in the therapeutic relationship takes place. When this happens the patient's risk may increase rapidly. Patients with BPD are sensitive to the clinician's perception of them and readily feel abandoned or become infected by hopelessness or become terrified that the clinician is going to end treatment because he or she cannot bear them. We are not suggesting that during SCM the clinician admits a patient to hospital for such reasons, instead more we recommend that such feelings indicate that reappraisal of treatment needs to take place and the level of risk of the patient carefully assessed by the treatment team (Colson et al., 1986). Most importantly the clinician needs to discuss the events within the team structure (see Chapter 3) and with an experienced clinician.

Fear and anxiety in the clinician as an indicator of increased risk should not be underestimated. Also, a clinician who cannot sleep at night because of worry about a patient is not an effective clinician, nor is a clinician who is fearful about letting a patient go home at the end of a meeting. Once a clinician recognizes that she is anxious about a patient and has tried to address this during the session but without success she should seek another opinion whenever possible. The aim is always to share the responsibility with the patient rather than taking over responsibility.

A related clinical situation may arise in which the clinician believes that she is necessary to keep a patient alive and so continues to see a patient for this reason rather than to increase the patient's interpersonal capacities and ability to manage emotional states. This situation is often explained by clinicians as arising from the powerful attachment relationship they have with the patient; nothing could be further from the truth. A relationship that is based on mutual clinging, with death as the organizing factor, is an adhesive relationship with no constructive reciprocity. It is unchangeable and pathologically rigid, and may need a structural intervention so that the clinician can be freed from fear. As a last resort hospital admission may be one of the potentially helpful interventions but discussion with a team or supervisor is best initially.

Hospital admission

Admitting a patient with BPD to the acute psychiatric ward is more than the practicalities of arranging the admission. The purpose of the admission has to be defined carefully, the ward program organized to meet the agreed aims, the staff appraised of the terms of the admission, plans made to monitor the progress, and arrangements made to integrate the continuing SCM program (NICE, 2009). Beware of setting unattainable targets for the patient. This will potentially engender despair in the patient and the staff when the goals are not achieved and even lead to early discharge against the patient's wishes, thereby increasing rather than decreasing the risk of suicide. Jointly with the patient, set aims that are in keeping with the work being done in the problem-solving group and individual sessions, and agree to a way of monitoring progress. The clinician liaises with the ward staff to ensure continuity of treatment and to help them manage any destructive behavior. If no progress on the BPD target problems occurs over a short time, for example a week, and there is no reduction in suicide risk for example, consider working on a discharge plan with the patient on the basis that the intervention of admission to an acute ward has not been beneficial (Bateman & Fonagy, 2006). A higher short-term risk approach may be necessary.

Overall the admission should be used to:

- stabilize the acute crisis—the patient wants to be understood at this point rather than to understand
- re-establish the care plan and crisis plan
- address changeable stressors
- reduce access to the means to suicide
- identify and mobilize current supports.

Prescribing in clinical practice

In this section we cover prescribing practice relevant to the implementation of SCM for BPD. There are two main sources informing prescribing practice for BPD, namely the guidelines promoted by the APA in the USA (Oldham, Phillips, Gabbard, & Soloff, 2001) and by NICE in the UK (NICE, 2009). Both offer somewhat distinct recommendations but share an emphatic warning about the dangers of overprescribing and lament equally the lack of evidence. The NICE guidance is based on data extracted from all the available studies on the use of medication at the time of publication. Subsequent meta-analytic studies of the evidence for the use of medication in BPD have given conflicting results (Lieb, Völlm, Rücker, Timmer, & Stoffers, 2010), but for the treatment of BPD in general psychiatric services we continue to recommend the guidance provided by NICE.

Summary of pharmacotherapy in BPD

Clinicians frequently offer medication to patients with BPD and the vast majority of patients, in desperation, accept it unquestioningly. Forty percent of patients with BPD take three or more medications concurrently, with 10% taking five or more (Zanarini, 2004). Given the intensity and extent of psychiatric symptoms experienced by people with BPD this fact is perhaps not surprising, but it is of considerable concern given the poor level of evidence for the use of drugs in the treatment of BPD. NICE guidelines found no evidence for the use of psychotropic medication and the Cochrane review came to similar conclusions; APA guidelines suggest that medications are primarily adjunctive to psychotherapy.

There have been about 28 placebo-controlled randomized controlled trials of the effectiveness of psychotropic medication in BPD. Initially selective serotonin reuptake inhibitors (SSRIs) were recommended for the treatment of mood, affective lability, emotion dysregulation, and anger and aggression partly because of the belief that BPD was related to mood disorders. However, current meta-analyses and systematic reviews find greater, albeit limited, support for antipsychotic (both typical and atypical) drugs as well as mood stabilizer medications for many of the symptoms associated with BPD, with decreasing evidence for the use of SSRIs unless there is a current comorbid major depressive episode (Abraham & Calabrese, 2008; Nose, Cipriani, Biancosino, Grassi, & Barbui, 2006; Ingenhoven, Lafay, Rinne, Passchier, & Duivenvoorden, 2010; Saunders & Silk, 2009; Stoffers et al., 2010).

So what is the clinician to do? The most important distinction is probably between prescribing medication as treatment for the constellation of symptoms that make up BPD, that is, treating that disorder itself, and recommending medication for comorbid or closely associated disorders—the former should be avoided whilst the latter may be given careful consideration if done within the context of a long-term treatment plan. Clinicians have long been guided by the idea that it was possible to divide the symptoms of personality disorder into those related to affect dysregulation, those suggesting impulse-behavioral dyscontrol, and those indicating cognitive–perceptual disturbance (Oldham et al., 2004). This may have some heuristic value but there is limited evidence that it predicts treatment response to different classes of medication. Nevertheless having BPD disrupts the normal course and treatment response of most other psychiatric disorders and so is of particular importance to the clinician.

Evidence for SSRIs is sparse and indicates they should only be used for the affective symptoms of a comorbid depressive episode and not for impulsivity, aggression or anxiety, although it has been suggested that fluvoxamine may reduce mood lability (Ingenhoven et al., 2010; Stoffers et al., 2010). Antipsychotic medication may help paranoid symptoms but it equally may improve affective lability as well as global functioning and overall psychopathology, suggesting a nonspecific effect (Silk & Jibson, 2010).

Mood stabilizers continue to be prescribed for patients despite their toxicity partly because there are open as well as placebo-controlled studies to support the use of divalproex sodium as well as placebo-controlled trials for topiramate and lamotrigine. Mood stabilizers seem most effective against impulsivity, aggression, anger/hostility, and interpersonal sensitivity (Abraham & Calabrese, 2008; Ingenhoven et al., 2010). There are methodological difficulties in randomized controlled trials involving lithium.

Other medication has been tried with naltrexone (for dissociative symptoms) (Bohus et al., 1999) and omega-3 fatty acids (for aggression and depression) (Zanarini & Frankenburg 2003) showing positive results.

In conclusion most classes of psychotropic medication appear to be effective to a limited degree for different symptoms of BPD (Lieb et al., 2010; NICE, 2009). As we mentioned in Chapter 1 there seems to be a shift towards using antipsychotics and/or mood stabilizers for many of these symptoms (Abraham & Calabrese, 2008), but the use of SSRIs is still popular with clinicians working in daily practice. More research using larger number of subjects for longer periods of time and using better consistency in outcome measures across studies needs to be undertaken.

Clinician cautions

Clinicians working in general psychiatric services need to take into account a number of pressures when prescribing for patients with personality disorder. These are of two types (Tyrer & Bateman, 2004). First, there are external factors. Clinicians may be asked to prescribe for patients by other mental health professionals and by general practitioners, when the indications are limited or even absent. In addition patients themselves may ask for medication not only in the hope that it might give a "quick fix" but also in their desperation to manage painful emotions. Second, there are internal factors related to the prescriber. Prescribers may feel that they have to prescribe even though symptoms likely to respond to medication are few and they will prescribe despite the absence of good evidence for the use of a specific drug in the treatment of BPD. Under these circumstances the clinician is more likely to prescribe either to manage a crisis or because of her own anxiety than for a patient's obvious benefit. Worse still the clinician justifies prescribing on specious grounds, for example maintaining that the symptoms for which they are prescribing are those of a comorbid disorder. Finally, they continue prescribing even though there has been no positive response to medication and despite evidence of harmful effects.

Fearful that we sound negative and judgmental about prescribers, we should now state at the outset that we mention these aspects of prescriber behavior bluntly because they need some explanation. Why would a clinician prescribe when the indications are limited and the research evidence is so poor? We will comment on this as we outline some prescribing guidance.

Prescribing guidance

When medication is used, it should always be considered in the context of a longer-term treatment plan; prescribing should be integrated into the overall management of the patient, not separated from but informed by the current context of clinical management.

Crisis

Medication is commonly started when a patient presents in crisis. This is often inevitable but is also the first error. Patients with BPD are regular users of psychiatric and acute hospital emergency services. Whilst there is no evidence for the use of specific medication in the crisis management of patients with BPD (NICE, 2009), professionals are hard-pressed and do not have time to initiate a psychological intervention. In line with patient demand and the level of patient distress, clinicians want to find a quick solution and the judicious use of medication may appear to offer an answer. However, whenever possible the psychiatric emergency clinician should limit the use of medication. It is better to discuss the crisis plan with the patient and contact the case manager to make an urgent appointment the following working day. This, of course, requires good coordination between services and between treatment staff and emergency staff. If the crisis presentation is during working hours the case manager should be contacted urgently for advice. The case manager can relay aspects of the crisis plan that are relevant.

Case manager

The case manager needs to follow certain principles, all of which are in keeping with the clinician general strategies discussed in Chapter 4, when discussing matters with a patient in the immediacy of a crisis. Most importantly, the case manager needs to revisit the crisis plan if it has been ineffective in the current context and needs redeveloping. It is also possible that the patient has not been able to follow her crisis plan and this needs investigation.

In revisiting the crisis plan the clinician should:

- maintain a relaxed and nonthreatening attitude
- use empathic open questioning and clarifying and validating statements to identify the onset and the course of the current problems
- try to understand the crisis from the point of view of the patient
- identify what aspects of the crisis plan the patient has tried
- explore the patient's reasons for distress
- seek to stimulate reflection about solutions and later additions or deletions from the crisis plan.

The clinician should not:

- minimize the stated reasons for the crisis
- offer solutions before full clarification of the problems
- challenge the patient excessively.

Finally, the clinician refers the patient back to the program of SCM and encourages further discussion of the problems in the prearranged individual meetings and the problem-solving group.

The prescriber

When considering drug treatment during crises, clinicians should whenever possible avoid adding medication to current prescriptions, thereby avoiding polypharmacy. What is more difficult to avoid is the second context for error, namely the prescriber's anxiety.

In a crisis, the psychiatrist or nurse prescriber may herself find it difficult to process her feelings and therefore reach for the prescription pad in a desire to "rescue" the patient or in a vain attempt to "do something." A patient who is suicidal may become emotionally demanding, leading to the psychiatrist being uncertain of what to do, which in turn makes her prescribe or decide to admit the patient to hospital. These reactions may account for the high number of medications prescribed to patients with BPD over time and the frequent number of hospital admissions. Zanarini found that at 2, 4, and 6 years after an index hospitalization 90% of her sample of patients with BPD were taking at least three medications at each time point (Zanarini, 2004; Zanarini, et al., 2003).

In order to minimize the adverse effects on prescribing which may result from the reactions of the prescriber to a patient's emotional states in a crisis, the clinician is referred back to Chapter 4 on clinician general strategies. There and in Chapter 3 we discuss the use of medication and its importance as an element of the initial crisis plan (see section on stabilizing medication in Chapter 3). Pharmacotherapy and the responsibilities of physicians during a crisis will have been discussed at the outset of treatment and this should be revisited. Some patients place an advanced directive statement in their crisis plan that even if they demand increases in medication during a crisis, the clinician should not give in to their demands unless there are over-riding medical reasons. The psychiatrist should not act unilaterally but work with the patient and the patient's current mental state, exploring this in relation to recent interpersonal events or difficulties in treatment. The psychiatrist can help find other ways of reducing the high level of anxiety or anger, the commonest emotions at crisis presentation.

Maintenance prescribing

Many patients with BPD take medication intermittently, fail to follow prescribing guidance, and may use prescribed medication in overdose when in crisis. These facts alone suggest that prescribing needs to be done carefully and preferably within the context of a trusting therapeutic relationship with a psychiatrist whose appointments are integrated into the treatment plan.

The potential beneficial effects and adverse effects of medication need to be discussed with patients prior to prescribing, the target symptoms clearly identified, an agreement made about how long a drug is to be used, and a method established to monitor the effect of the drug on symptoms. Most important is the patient's agreement to take medication in the first place. The initial role of the doctor is to provide information and to remain reasonably neutral about whether the patient takes medication or not, since a patient bullied into taking a drug is not likely adhere to the prescribing guidance. Conversely, a prescriber who is bullied into giving medication needs to be aware that resentment or other feelings might interfere with her adherence to effective prescribing. Remaining neutral is not the same as declining to give a recommendation for a specific drug for an explicit reason such as targeting distressing and persistent symptoms. After information has been given to the patient, the prescriber may make a recommendation but should not become overly engaged in persuading the patient to follow advice. The more a prescriber attempts to convince a patient to take a drug the greater the patient's resistance may be, the more it undermines clinician–patient collaboration, and the more it undermines promoting patient self-capabilities and belief in their capabilities.

There is no evidence that patients with personality disorder need higher doses of medication than other patients. Dosage should be kept within the normal therapeutic range. The clinician should bear in mind that the evidence suggests that patients with BPD may receive inappropriate combinations and be prescribed excessive numbers of psychotropic medications at any one time (Sansone, Rytwinski, & Gaither, 2003). Any patient, whatever their current diagnosis, who describes a treatment history of polypharmacy with limited beneficial response should have their diagnosis reviewed with consideration given to the possibility of a diagnosis of BPD.

Some patients may seek quick results, yet the effects of medication may take some time to become apparent, so it is necessary to warn the patients of a likely delay so that medication will not be stopped early. The best way to do this is to take an interest in how the patient responds to the medication and to arrange regular meetings to discuss symptom change, side-effects, and changes in dose. An appropriately skilled case manager instead of the psychiatrist can do this as long as their work is well coordinated.

Time on medication

In general patients should expect to take medication for a minimum of 2–4 weeks unless there are intolerable side-effects, and this principle is best agreed when medication is started. If the patient stops a drug unilaterally before the agreed time, it is best not to prescribe other medication until the 2–4 week period is completed. This reduces the demand for drug after drug when no effect occurs within a few days and prevents "creeping" polypharmacy. Soloff and colleagues (Soloff, Cornelius, & George, 1993) have suggested that an exception to this type of rule is antipsychotic medication such as haloperidol, when the benefits may occur rapidly but wane within a few weeks. Discontinuation may therefore be appropriate after a few weeks. Discontinuation of medication needs to be done carefully and many clinicians believe that patients with BPD, whilst more prone to placebo responsiveness (Soloff et al., 1993), are also more sensitive to the side-effects and withdrawal effects of medication than other patients, although there is little evidence that this is the case; nevertheless reducing medication slowly whilst implementing another is probably the safest course.

Zanarini (Zanarini et al., 2012; Zanarini, Frankenburg, Reich, & Fitzmaurice, 2010b) demonstrated that at 16-year follow-up people with BPD are as likely to have died from other causes as died from suicide, with many of these other causes being obesity related. Given the recognized role of psychotropic medications in contributing to obesity, the prescriber will need to keep this long-term view in mind when considering prescribing and the duration of prescribing (Frankenburg & Zanarini, 2006).

As we have indicated, maintaining sensible rules is harder than it sounds because patient demand and clinician judgment are influenced by transference and countertransference phenomena. The psychiatrist is not immune from countertransference responses even if her task is solely to look after medication.

Comorbid conditions

Now we come to the third pitfall in prescribing for people with BPD. Prescribing should be limited to treatment of comorbid conditions and not given to patients for symptoms of BPD itself (NICE, 2009). The prescriber must try to differentiate between comorbid disorders and BPD. A number of indicators help to differentiate the two. Symptoms with sudden onset, which are responsive to environmental triggers and primarily related to relationship problems, or have obvious link to managing varying anxiety, and which fluctuate in intensity and predominance, are more likely to be part of BPD than, say, an underlying depressive disorder. Persistence and pervasiveness of symptoms should alert the clinician to a possible comorbid disorder which needs further investigation.

Finally

The following practice guidance based on NICE guidance (NICE, 2009) may help the clinician when prescribing for comorbid conditions in the context of BPD.

The drug used should:

♦ target specific symptoms of the comorbid condition
♦ have minimum side-effects
♦ have low addictive properties
♦ show minimal potential for abuse
♦ be relatively safe in overdose.

The doctor and patient need to:

♦ ensure that there is consensus about medication between themselves and the case manager and other involved professionals, and identify the primary prescriber
♦ agree on the target symptoms
♦ jointly agree a plan for adherence
♦ avoid polypharmacy
♦ agree on regular prescriptions of fewer tablets at a time, depending on risk
♦ monitor response carefully
♦ discontinue a drug after a trial period if there is no response
♦ consider if additional or further psychological intervention is required
♦ ensure that prescription is not used to avoid implementing other more appropriate interventions
♦ consider the relationship between patient and therapist as part of the context of prescribing, e.g. be aware that prescribing may be used primarily to signify care.

Chapter 7

Family and friends

Summary

- ◆ Why include family/friends in treatment?
  - • Family often live with and financially and emotionally support the person with BPD.
  - • Family members of people with BPD experience high levels of distress and burden.
  - • Otherwise the person with BPD merely returns to the same environment where behaviors have been maintained.
  - • Higher family involvement has been predictive of better outcomes.
- ◆ We have arbitrarily broken down interventions into short (two-session) and multisession formats for ease of discussion.
- ◆ A two-session intervention is feasible for time-strapped generalist mental health clinicians.
- ◆ A two-session intervention might include:
  - • assessment
  - • accurate information on BPD
  - • support
  - • validation
  - • nonblaming causal explanation of BPD
  - • realistic hope
  - • orientation to treatment
  - • psychoeducation on reinforcement
  - • encouragement of self-care
  - • provision of suitable reading
  - • advising where to find family/friends support groups.
- ◆ Multisession interventions can be of varied duration and take a number of formats.

- Suitable family/friends reading resources are provided.
- Valuable, albeit modest, research exists of the effectiveness of a number of multisession family/friends formats.
- A brief BPD information handout for families and friends is provided as an appendix for readers who might want to give this to family and friends.

Family/friend comment

I have two messages for clinicians:
1. BPD is treatable.
2. If we can't get to BPD specialists, some of the specialized knowledge needs to get to generalist clinicians.

This book is based wherever possible on evidence. Whilst there are some studies of family and friend interventions in specialist settings, there are not yet any evidence-based studies of family and friend interventions in generalist mental health settings. The manuals of the four studies discussed in Chapter 2 provide just a small amount of information about family interventions used (SCM for adults involves family members in the assessment; GCC for adolescents actively engages families in assessment, psychoeducation, treatment planning and provision of support, and up to four sessions of family therapy). As authors we were therefore left in a quandary whether to write a chapter about family and friend involvement, deciding in the end that the area was clinically important and, despite the absence of research in generalist mental health settings, would nevertheless be welcomed by most general readers. Although there are no studies of family involvement in generalist settings, the modest research in specialist settings (which is provided at the end of the chapter), has guided our suggestions in this chapter.

In this chapter we provide an introduction and sections on:

- level of family involvement
- guiding suggestions for short two-session interventions for time-restricted clinicians
- brief comments for multisession interventions where resources exist
- summary of the research data

We have generally used the language of "family/friends" to indicate that our focus is on family and friends, but of course partners and even closely involved employers are included. However, on some occasions where this language use becomes overly cumbersome we have opted for using just "family" to refer to family, friends and others closely involved with the person with BPD. Both clinician and patient need to decide who to invite to "family and friend" meetings. On one occasion the clinician and patient invited the other members of a rock band that the patient played in as they were the patient's closest emotional ties.

Most of our comments are directed towards family and friends of adults with BPD. Where an adolescent has BPD, involving family members embedded into the treatment package is even more important. Early intervention for adolescents with BPD is increasingly being encouraged by experts working with adolescents. Early intervention is likely to be more effective before problematical patterns get locked in.

Introduction

The UK NICE guidelines outline the rationale for involving families in the treatment of BPD extremely well (NICE, 2009). They state:

+ If the service user agrees, carers (who may include family and friends) should have the opportunity to be involved in decisions about treatment and care. Families and carers should also be given the information and support they need.
+ When a person is diagnosed with BPD, the effect of the diagnosis on carers is often overlooked. (p. 101)
+ Carers of people with BPD may have needs that are at least equivalent to carers of people with other severe and enduring mental health problems. (p. 102)
+ ... emerging evidence suggests that structured family programmes may be helpful ... ' (p. 103)
+ Further research is needed to build on the emerging evidence suggesting that structured psychoeducation programmes that also facilitate social support networks may be helpful for families.

Why include family/friends in treatment?

+ Family members often live with, and financially and emotionally support, the person with BPD.
+ Family members of people with BPD experience high levels of distress and burden.

- ◆ Otherwise the person with BPD merely returns to same environment where behaviors have been maintained.
- ◆ Higher family involvement has been predictive of better outcomes.

(Pirkis et al., 2012)

Family/friend comment

Part of the frustration family members experience is the result of emotionally and financially dealing with numerous diagnoses and treatments before the family member ever receives a BPD diagnosis, and ultimately not having adequate treatment and support systems available. It also does not make sense to treat the person with BPD in isolation, with them just returning back to the same unchanged environment where their behaviors developed and/or continue.

It is well recognized that the family of people with mental illness experience high levels of distress and burden (McFarlane, Dixon, Lukens, & Lucksted, 2003), including financial stress (costs incurred, loss of earnings due to care-giving role). Family/friends of people with BPD report difficulty accessing accurate information about BPD, wrestle with a healthcare system that stigmatizes them, struggle with hopelessness, financial stress, and reduced social networks (Buteau, Dawkins, & Hoffman, 2008), and have high levels of chronic stress and strained relationships (Giffin, 2008).

Family/friend comment

It took numerous misdiagnoses (including BPD not even being mentioned as a possibility), hundreds of futile prescriptions, tens of thousands of dollars, and 3 years to finally arrive at a BPD diagnosis of my daughter. On the one hand it was a relief to finally get what I believe was the correct diagnosis; on the other hand the lack of public information about the disorder was extremely frustrating. After the psychiatrist's brief explanation about the disorder, we went scurrying to the library and bookstores in vain trying to find out as much as we could that would help us "deal" with our daughter and get her the help she needed.

Couples that include a person with BPD have high levels of relationship difficulties, including breakups and reconciliations (Bouchard, Sabourin, Lussier, & Villeneuve, 2009; Whisman & Schonbrun, 2009), and substantial risk of violence (Newhill, Eack, & Mulvey, 2009; Zanarini et al., 1999). Much has been written about how challenging it is for us as professionals to work with people with BPD and consequently the need for us to be well trained and supported in this work in order to be effective and not burn out. Whilst we as professionals might spend 1 hour a week with the person with BPD, family members frequently live together 24/7. Despite this, there has been limited recognition of the difficulties and challenges faced by family members and little in the way of supporting and assisting family/friends with specific skills. Also, without sharing basic knowledge and skills with family members, the person with BPD merely returns each week after treatment to the same environment where their behaviors were maintained. As general mental health clinicians we can change this. In our experience, family/friends who attend sessions with clinicians are thirsty for support, skills, and reading material written expressly for them. Most educational support groups and reading materials are typically targeted to people with Axis I diagnoses, thus BPD families have to search long and hard to have their needs met.

Family/friend comment

We need reading materials that are specifically about BPD. I don't think that this can be stressed enough. Finding these on our own can be a long journey with endless dead-ends that can put off all but the most determined of family members.

There are numerous randomized controlled trials demonstrating the effectiveness of family psychoeducation interventions provided by professionals on reducing relapses for schizophrenia (McFarlane et al., 2003) and also with depression and substance use. The most well-known community-based family education program run by families for families is the National Alliance on Mental Illness's "Family-to-family" program (Dixon et al., 2004), which covers a range of Axis I conditions and is reported by Hoffman and Fruzzetti (2007). The different needs of families of people with BPD and the person with BPD have led to the development of more BPD-focused family interventions, a summary of the results of which are outlined at the end of the chapter.

Family/friend comment

Education and support groups for families of people with mental illness were helpful, however whilst schizophrenia, bipolar disorder and depression were frequently named, BPD was not even mentioned. Later, we really got our needs met in groups that were specifically for families and friends of people with BPD.

Family member involvement

"Expressed emotion" is a construct describing relationships characterized by high involvement, criticism, and hostility. High "expressed emotion" has been shown to be a strong predictor of outcome for people with mood disorders and eating disorders (Butzlaff & Hooley, 1998). For people with schizophrenia, it has been shown that a high level of family member involvement in the context of high "expressed emotion" predicts poorer outcomes for the person with schizophrenia (Brown, Birley, & Wing, 1972; Kuipers, 1979; Leff, Kuipers, Berkowitz, Eberlein-Vries, & Sturgeon, 1982; Vaughn & Leff, 1976). In the area of BPD, exactly the opposite has been shown to be the case (Hoffman & Hooley, 1998; Hooley & Hoffman, 1999), with high family member involvement predicting better outcomes (especially lower re-hospitalization) amongst people with BPD. Contrary to initial expectations, family member criticism and hostility did not predict outcome (Hooley & Hoffman, 1999). This is highly clinically relevant information for generalist mental health professionals and for family members. Hooley and Hoffman (1999) postulate that high involvement of family members may be received by the person with BPD as a "signal" that "the family cares" and recognizes their suffering without minimizing or ignoring it. Hence the involvement may be experienced as validating. Hooley and Hoffman (1999) suggest that a high level of involvement may address abandonment concerns as this "may provide a great deal of reassurance that there is someone in their life who will remain with them for the long-term." From the data that higher family involvement predicted better outcomes for people with BPD, Hoffman, Fruzzetti, and Buteau (2007) suggest that "borderline patients need the involvement of family as long as emotional validation accompanies any criticism or hostility."

Family/friend comment

Why don't clinicians involve the family—perhaps because they are concerned that if the door is cracked open a little, family members might come barging in and the clinician ends up treating an entire family instead of one patient. But based on Hooley and Hoffman's study, rather than being viewed as part of the problem, educated and involved family members can be viewed as part of the solution or treatment. In this way, involving family members can decrease rather than increase the work of clinicians—and allow clinicians the pleasure of seeing a number of satisfied people.

Guidance on how mental health professionals can involve family/friends

How might a generalist mental health clinician involve family/friends in their work? The quantitative outcome research outlined at the end of this chapter, whilst limited, demonstrates that, in general, engaging with families can be productive for the person with BPD and/or productive for family/friends. Salient points from this outcome research can then be synthesized with the qualitative research from family members providing guidance for us as generalist mental health clinicians.

We wish to acknowledge that there are situations where a close family/friend has been the perpetrator of significant past abuse, or worse still where the abuse is continuing to occur. It is our experience that generally in these situations the person with BPD does not want this family/friend involved or the family/friend does not want to be involved or both. Where abuse is current and ongoing, attending to safety factors is the highest priority and couple or family/friends interventions, if engaged in, might best be done after working with the victim of the abuse to ensure their safety first. Sometimes, partners are involved in unilateral or bilateral physical or verbal abuse, with both parties wanting the abuse to end. In these situations the couple often do want to, and are often desperately keen to, attend sessions with mental health professionals.

There are situations when the person with BPD and the mental health professional choose not to involve family/friends. Alongside these situations, we need to respond to the research that a high level of family involvement is statistically predictive of a better outcome for the person with BPD and respond to the research of positive outcomes for family-focused interventions. In clinical practice we therefore want to involve family/friends enthusiastically and frequently, whilst leaving a space for occasionally not involving those where involvement is assessed as being counterproductive or at least counterproductive at that point.

We have arbitrarily broken down interventions into two-session and multisession formats for ease of discussion. This could also be conceptualized as short and medium duration interventions. The tasks outlined in two-session interventions can of course be carried out over several sessions, where time permits and need is present. Given the research evidence of effectiveness of multisession family/friends interventions, where resources exist, as general mental health clinicians we need either to provide or refer family/friends members to these resources. This will be briefly discussed later, but first, what do we do where these multisession resources do not exist?

Short intervention (two sessions or more)

In the common situation for generalist mental health professionals where resources for multisession interventions of families is not possible, a short two-session intervention of families can have a huge impact and be time efficient and effective.

The Hoffman and Hooley (1999) study demonstrating improved outcomes with a high level of family involvement provides evidence to counter the historical situation of family members being criticized, stigmatized or at worst vilified for having a child with BPD. This research evidence is important to share with those family members where ongoing abuse is not occurring.

Where clinicians value family contact highly and have decided that meeting with family is not contraindicated, it is our experience that most clients with BPD welcome or at least tolerate a short two-session meeting of clinician and client with BPD and family.

In a two-session intervention we can:

- validate the huge challenges family/friends face—in our experience this can be a defining experience for family members who up until that moment have often been the subject of criticism and blame for their family members' condition

- provide accurate information about BPD, including diagnosis

- provide realistic hope based on BPD prognosis and treatment outcome studies

- where applicable, provide a nonblaming plausible theory of causality

- orient family/friends to the treatment that will be provided, including roles of therapy, medication, crisis services, and hospitalization

- use orientation to proactively decrease the likelihood of polarizations occurring between the person with BPD, family/friends, and the treating clinician/organization—in this way all parties are more likely to be pulling together

- provide information on what to do if the person with BPD self-harms or has urges to suicide, and whom to communicate with

- support family/friends by linking them with family/friends in similar positions to their own. Many cities have some form of general mental health family member support and education groups. The Family Connections program offered by the National Education Alliance for BPD (NEA-BPD) specifically for families of people with BPD is now available in a number of geographical areas (in the USA in particular and also other countries) and recently a US teleconferencing version has been developed and used in the USA for those living outside areas that run face-to-face programs.

◆ affirm the legitimacy of looking after oneself

◆ provide suitable family/friends specific reading material

◆ provide a list of further reading material

◆ assess the suitability of doing or referring for multisession family/friends intervention

◆ time permitting provide psychoeducation about validation skills, including what we know has worked for other family/friends from research and teach validation skills.

Family/friend comment

Encourage "positive grieving!" People need very much to tell their stories. It is so very sad that often people are not available who can listen to and cope with stories of burden, grief, and trauma that permeate the family system when BPD is present, or that family and friends are just too embarrassed to tell anyone else. The story of the ongoing pain in our hearts is simply not the small talk we share with our neighbor over the back fence, or at the office while standing around the water cooler. So the importance of you listening to us and helping us to find one another so that we might share our stories together in a group is of great value. The process of sharing seems to have a healing effect both on the teller of the story and on those who are hearing it.

"Positive grieving" is a time when family members' pain and suffering can be acknowledged and their efforts validated by others. It is a time to listen with deep respect and empathy about the obstacles families face at every turn—about home life in chaos—perhaps for many years, of the estrangement of families, of the loss of friends and social life. If symptoms started early, how few resources were available within the school system to help with raising the child, and how often school staff blamed the parenting of the child, particularly the mother. How hard it was to confide in anyone! Many a school nurse, pediatrician, or GP have not understood or even believed symptoms to be occurring.

And in the USA, where we don't yet have universal health care, of life savings gone, of homes mortgaged, all spent seeking care for a beloved relative, usually a child. The ramifications of the impact of this condition on the family can reverberate back to the relative with BPD, so that family members with their own levels of depression and distress may be less available to their relative with BPD. Educating family and friends about the disorder, welcoming us, and recognizing us for who we really are (lay partners in treatment) can have a positive impact on our well-being.

Family/friend comment

The natural course of BPD is that people generally improve over time. As a mother who has come repeatedly, perilously close to losing my child to suicide, I encourage you, amongst other things, to look to "buy time" in which contact is maintained by you not just at times of crisis but longitudinally over time. What I am suggesting is, provided your client is willing, that you keep track of your BPD clients who drop out of treatment by staying in contact with them through a mailed letter inquiring of their well-being, say four times per year for at least 2 years. This indicates that as their clinician you have not abandoned them, even when they have walked out on you. I believe that act of willing contact from you would be helpful to family members who are often holding the fort by themselves.

Critical step of etiological understandings for family members

Understanding the cause of BPD can be a critical watershed point for many family members and might well be the single most important intervention that time-strapped general mental health clinicians can provide for family members. As mentioned earlier, family members have often been subject to criticism and blame for supposedly causing BPD in their loved one. In addition, as probably a majority of parents would do, family members often experience intense guilt about having been unable to parent their child into an adulthood that they had envisaged. Of course, as any parent would, parents have been reaching for understandings of how their loved one got to develop BPD and what contributions they as parents might have made.

For all these reasons, parents will often arrive at sessions with huge feelings of guilt and burden. In addition to the obvious suffering involved, intense burden and guilt restricts the capacity for all of us, including family, to learn new skills. Family are searching for an understanding of cause that fits with their lived experience, is realistic, and has depth. A causal understanding, which acknowledges the pain and suffering of all parties and the realistic contributions that the person with BPD and the family members may have made whilst not blaming either party, is crucial.

Whilst etiological factors have been covered in Chapter 1, they are briefly summarized again here with an emphasis on family member perspectives. Most leading international researchers and clinicians in the field are in agreement that biological and psychological factors can contribute to the development of the condition and that there is often a transactional interplay between these biological and psychological factors. Biological research findings associated with BPD (e.g., sluggish serotonin system, smaller amygdala and hippocampus, altered pre-frontal lobe functioning) and genetic factors (twin studies, DNA studies) shared in lay language can be experienced by family members as validating and supportive. Family are likely to feel validated by Porr's use of the metaphors of the amygdala being the brain's emotional gas pedal (overactive in BPD), the pre-frontal cortex being the brain's emotional brake (underactive in BPD), and serotonin (sluggish in BPD) being the brain system's oil (Porr, 2010).

We can share research demonstrating the increased recognition of a substantial genetic contribution to personality. Having a particular gene has been associated with a five-fold increase in the rate of self-harm behavior (Joyce et al., 2006). Data from twin studies demonstrate genetic contributions to BPD of 30–50% (Bornovalova et al., 2009) with Distel et al.'s study (Distel et al., 2008) demonstrating the same genetic contributions (42%) across three countries (The Netherlands, Belgium, Australia). Genetic factors may manifest as personality traits such as emotion intensity, sensitivity, and reactivity, impulsivity, irritability, and novelty-seeking. One large study of identical and nonidentical twins of people with BPD showed that the identical twins had a five times increased chance of having BPD compared to nonidentical twins (Torgersen et al., 2000).

We need to be mindful that some family members may experience guilt about the genetic contribution to the disorder. However, in our experience, burden and guilt about genetic contributions are usually more than offset by the decreased guilt and burden experienced by a self-construct of not having been and not being a "bad" parent.

DBT theory is that people with BPD may be born experiencing emotion more intensely (emotionally sensitive and reactive) than the rest of the population, which is neither inherently positive nor negative. Parents of children with BPD describe problems as early as infancy compared to their other children or other children that they know who did not develop BPD (Goodman et al., 2010). Sharing this theory with family members can be validating and affirming of parents' experience of the difficulty of parenting such a person who may often be temperamentally different from themselves. That is, it would be difficult for any parent to parent a child who has a temperament that the parent has no experience of, and even more difficult when this temperament is of high emotional sensitivity ("poorness of fit") (Fruzzetti, Shenk, & Hoffman, 2005). The quality of the parenting received might well have been sufficient for other children born less emotionally sensitive but was unfortunately insufficient for the person born emotionally sensitive. So, the sad situation here is that even the most caring of parents may be unable to teach their child how to work with, manage, and celebrate their intense emotions. If this happens, the child may feel misunderstood, which will then impact on the parents, who may feel ineffective at parenting and misunderstood; a cycle of misunderstanding may become embedded. We have seen parents and their adult children in tears of joy (and sadness of lost years) on hearing and discussing this explanation of cause, shifting to a position of neither parents nor adult child being to blame, with each party having done the best they knew how. This can set the stage for all parties to move on to solutions in the present and future.

We find discussion about attachment relationships frees up the families once they realize that disruption in the attachment bond has many causes and can occur with one child but not another. A temperamentally sensitive and reactive child can disrupt the formation of a secure bond between the child and parent with both the child and parents becoming anxious, which impacts on further development, however hard the parent tries to change things. This is the "poorness of fit" which sensitizes the child to other events, for example at school with peers, which would otherwise not be harmful. We also discuss changes in neurobiology that can occur during development that interact with the attachment process and lead to problems of mentalizing over time. Parents rapidly identify with the experience that their child misunderstands their motives and characterizes them in ways that are alien to themselves.

Being brought up in an environment that was abusive or neglectful will obviously have a profound impact on our psychological development, decreasing our chances of entering adulthood with psychological skills, good self-esteem, and confidence. Widom and colleagues (2009) report an increased risk of BPD 30 years later in a prospective study of children with court-documented physical abuse or neglect. People with childhood sexual abuse when followed up are five times more likely to self-harm as adults (Joyce et al., 2006). People with BPD report a high incidence of sexual abuse (40–70%). It is our experience that where a history of physical and/or sexual abuse exists, family member/s who are willingly engaged with their child and the child's mental health services are invariably not the perpetrator/s of the abuse. It is important to remember also that in at least 30% and perhaps up to 60%, a history of sexual abuse is not present.

Family/friend comment

It is my experience in running family support and education groups for family of people with BPD that those of us who are continuing to be involved in our adult child's lives are not perpetrators of abuse or neglect. We struggle enormously with the burden of association and hope that clinicians will see us for who we are; concerned and often struggling parents who are not abusers.

Family/friend comment

My most important message to clinicians is to include the "poorness-of-fit" concept in the two-session intervention, and make sure you save time to teach and practice validation skills.

Provide realistic hope

Family members have stated that they would like clinicians to respond to the frequent hopelessness that they face (Buteau et al., 2008). It is easy to see how the often slow rate of change in people with BPD plus family/friends' common feelings of intense anguish and powerlessness, leads to a sense of hopelessness. Fortunately, as clinicians we have access to longitudinal prognosis and treatment outcome data that demonstrate that people in general do improve over time. We also need to compassionately acknowledge the very real risk of suicide, where, of course, the statistically positive outcome of BPD in general would be irrelevant to family/friends that might lose someone dear to them. Familiarity with the McLean Study of Adult Development (MSAD) that demonstrated that 86% of people with BPD had had a remission of BPD of greater than 4 years at 10-year follow-up (Zanarini et al., 2006, 2010b), will be most helpful to share with family/friends members concerned that their loved one will never improve or recover. This naturalistic improvement over time appears to be considerably speeded up by receiving effective evidence-based treatments. As we have highlighted in this book, whilst specialist treatments are highly desirable, there is now data that high-quality general treatments can also be substantially and statistically significantly effective.

Teach validation and empathy skills

Validation is a term that we see as being roughly equivalent to three-part empathy (empathic resonance, expressed empathy, and received empathy). By this definition one has to understand where the person is "at," communicate this understanding, and do it effectively enough so as to promote the person experiencing the intervention as validating or empathic. As such, validation is transactional with an inherent built in feedback loop. Validation is a skill for family/friends to use that is drawn from the research of what has worked for other family/friends, is the skill that we think is of most clinical relevance for time strapped generalist mental health clinicians to teach families, and is the single skill that we would focus on teaching family members if time allowed in a short two-session intervention. We would only mention this skill once family members have felt validated and empathized with themselves (including causal understanding), which helps them move away from blame and self-blame to solutions. Suggesting that family members validate the person with BPD before they have themselves felt validated (including around etiology) could well be experienced as invalidating and unempathic. We also name the universal value of validation skills for optimal relationships for all of us, not just for families of people with BPD.

As generalist clinicians, we can provide a definition of validation being when the other person "gets where one is coming from" and name what a great gift this is for anybody to receive—that is, to be seen for who we are and how we see ourselves. An important teaching point for family members is that validation is in the "eye of the beholder." That is, a comment or action made with the best of intentions to validate, which we consider validating, is only validating if the other person experiences the comment or action as validating. If one's attempts to validate are experienced as not validating, one can always apologize and try again, knowing that with a hyperemotionally sensitive person, one may fail more often than succeed in these efforts, at least initially—but making the effort can in itself be beneficial.

We can share that research has demonstrated the value of validation skills in enhancing family/friends well-being and perceptions of family/friends relationships (Fruzzetti & Iverson, 2006; Fruzzetti, Santisteban, & Hoffman, 2007; Hoffman et al., 2005, 2007; Rajalin, Wickholm-Pethrus, Hursti, & Jokinen, 2009). We can share research (which is likely to be consistent with family/friends personal experience of being validated) that validation results in decreased agitation in the person being validated. Decreased agitation results in increased capacity to be effective, including an improved capacity to accurately express experience, which in turn increases the likelihood of the other person being validating. This intervention breaks the previous transactional cycle of agitation, inaccurate expression of experience, invalidation, increased agitation, and so on (Fruzzetti et al., 2005, 2007; Fruzzetti, et al., 2005).

It will be important to emphasize that in many situations one might have to work hard at finding something valid to validate, what Linehan refers to using the metaphors of "the kernel of truth" or "the nugget of gold in a cup of sand"(Linehan, 1993b, p. 241). For example, we would not want to validate self-harm as a solution to distress, but can validate how distressed the person must have been to resort to self-harm.

It will also be important to share what is realistically achievable by validation in a single situation. Validation might defuse the situation like "pouring oil on troubled waters" but may take 10 minutes of repeated validation before having an effect. It might be that skilful validation does not have an impact at all; however, in these situations at least the person hasn't made things worse by "pouring petrol onto an already raging fire."

Feel free to share with family/friends and if appropriate give them a photocopy of the following description of validation by a person who benefitted from learning validation in a multifamily intervention.

I might have said that I feel really ugly and did not want to leave the house and previously my mother would have said that was exactly the reason that I should go out—face my fears. Whilst this had been true, because it was done on its own without also validating my experience, I had not been able to benefit from her well-meaning advice. Once we all learnt validation, my mother was able to step back and validate me by saying something like, "That must be terrible, feeling that way. Is there anything that I can do to help?" After a time of us all using validation with each other, it really opened up the commu-nication between me and my family/friends. They felt like they were helping me—and they were!(Krawitz, 2008)

DBT validation

We can share the way that DBT structures validation as follows:

V1: "Listening"—Listening like our life depends upon it. We can add that the viability of family relationships might well depend on "5 Gold Star" listening.

V2: "Accurate reflection"

V3: "Articulating the unverbalized"—We might give an example of seeing a person with head down saying very little, and asking the person whether they are feeling sad. We need to be sure to emphasize that as we are guessing what the other person is experiencing (they may after all be experiencing anxiety, guilt or shame), we need to put forward our guess tentatively and in an inquiring manner, ready to change if the person says, "No, I am not sad, I am … "

V4: "Normalizing" in the context of the person's biology and past experiences. For example, "It makes sense that you are anxious about this forthcoming situation, given how things have not worked out for you in the past."

V5: "Normalizing" in the context of the current situation. For example, "Most people would feel the way that you do if they were in the same situation, I certainly would." DBT values this V5 normalizing validation highly.

Practical validation: This refers to situations when doing what is required is better than using words. Examples may be passing tissues to someone who is crying or washing the dirty dishes for someone who is exhausted after a hard day.

Teaching mentalizing and mentalizing skills

We teach and rehearse some basic mentalizing skills with families. This can be done quite quickly once the concept has been explained in terms of understanding what is going on in other minds. Families find the idea of mentalizing links with a commonsense psychology and makes sense to them partly because they have felt so misunderstood by the person with BPD who may have, at times, misconstrued their motives. When considering how one mentalizes successfully in relation to other people's thought and emotions we distinguish between 12 distinct characteristics of relational strengths (Bateman & Fonagy, 2006). We do not necessarily cover all these but choose the ones that seem relevant to a particular family depending on the family interaction pattern they identify. We role play the family interaction using the specific attitudes.

(1) *Curiosity* (Cecchin, 1987) refers to an attitude where the individual is genuinely interested in other people's thoughts and emotions, and respectful of the perspectives of others. It includes an attitude of expectation that one's understanding will be elaborated or expanded by what is in another person's mind and it implies an openness to discovery and a reluctance to make assumptions, or hold prejudices, about what others think or feel.

(2) The *stance of safe uncertainty* (Mason, 1993)—also elsewhere referred to as *"the opaqueness of mental states"* (Leslie, 1987)—refers to the open acknowledgment that one can never know but only imagine or make an informed guess about what other people are thinking. It is "safe" in that this does not lead to the person becoming totally perplexed or overwhelmed by what may happen in the minds of others. This confidence is based on a background feeling that the reactions of others are at least to some extent predictable, given the sense one may have of what others may think and feel.

(3) *Reflective contemplation* is a mentalizing attitude which conveys a flexible, relaxed, and open approach rather than a controlled and compulsive pursuit of how others think and feel.

(4) *Perspective-taking* is characterized by the acceptance that the same phenomenon or process can look very different from different perspectives and that these tend to reflect the individuals' different experiences and histories.

(5) *Forgiveness* is a mentalizing strength which bases the comprehension of the actions of others on understanding and accepting their mental states. An example of this is the management, if not dissipation, of one's anger towards a person who has behaved offensively, once one has understood that the other person had acted as they did for a particular reason, such as a significant personal loss.

(6) *Impact awareness* is another important aspect of successful mentalizing. It refers to the appreciation of how one's own thoughts, emotions, and actions may affect others.

(7) *A trusting attitude* is seen as a mentalizing strength, since trust is at the core of secure attachment. Importantly, the opposite of a secure attachment is a paranoid, fearful stance (not some form of "nonattachment"), which is incompatible with mentalizing.

(8) *Humility* (moderation) in relation to one's capacity to know and understand someone else and willingness therefore to be surprised and learn from others regardless of status follows from many of the strengths described above.

(9) *Playfulness and (self-mocking) humor* may be an expression of humility and is a key component of the therapeutic mentalizing attitude.

(10) The *willingness to take turns* articulates an approach of "give and take" in interactions with family members and significant others. This includes the ability to make oneself available to be understood and taking an interest in extending one's understanding by taking in the other person's thoughts and preoccupations.

(11) The mentalizing stance implies a *belief in changeability* since minds *can* be changed, generally imbuing a sense of optimism into the family interaction.

(12) Finally, the intentional stance of mentalizing implies *assuming responsibility and accepting accountability* since one's actions are generated by one's own thoughts, emotions, wishes, beliefs, and desires, whether one is fully conscious of them at the time of the action or not.

Consumer comment

My parents came back from a meeting for families with BPD which I had refused to go to. As soon as I asked them what had been talked about, I sensed a change in their attitude. They explained what had been talked about and then wanted to know what I thought about it. Before, they would have said that I should have gone if I wanted to know what was talked about. But this time they even agreed that they would not interrupt me as they tried to get my point of view. They said they were trying to see things from my perspective. At first I was suspicious and thought that the whole thing was a trick of some sort. Then I thought that it was about time. But they insisted that their meeting had suggested that it could help them help me if they saw things from my point of view. It was then that I realized I had to change by trying to explain to them how I saw things. It is incredible how difficult this was.

Teach brief principles of positive reinforcement

We can provide brief psychoeducation about positive reinforcement, another universal skill for optimal psychological health and functioning, not just for families of people with BPD but for all of us, that includes the following points:

- A reinforcer is something that increases the likelihood of a desired behavior occurring again (e.g., "You did so well when you asserted yourself without yelling").

- A punisher is something aversive that decreases the likelihood of the desired behavior occurring again (e.g., "Because you yelled at me, I will not be driving you to the station; you will have to walk").

- Reinforcement is in general more effective than aversive punishment.

- Aversive punishment can stop behaviors occurring (e.g., yelling) but not promote new behaviors (e.g., how to express oneself when angry without yelling).

- Reinforcement can promote new behaviors (e.g., how to express oneself when angry without yelling).

- Reinforcers will be different for different people. For example, praise is commonly a reinforcer, but occasionally is experienced by some as aversive and actually decreases the likelihood of the behavior being repeated.

- Reinforcers work best when they occur immediately after the desired behavior.

- When desired behaviors are realistically out of reach, one can reinforce small successive approximations.

The most common reinforcers used and received in our lives whether we are a person with BPD, family member or clinician is the natural (vs contrived) interest, engagement, and verbal praise immediately following the event that is being reinforced. For example, "You did so well to manage your distress without self-harming."

Self-care

We believe that all human beings have a right to be on this planet and to strive for happiness. Family members have high rates of burden and deserve to look after themselves. Whilst there has not yet been published research on the impact on the person with BPD of healthy family members, we believe it to be likely that family members who look after themselves will actually have a positive spin-off effect on loved ones with whom they are in a relationship; as was demonstrated in a recent yet-to-be-published study of a "Family Connections" program for family and friends of people with BPD. Looking after oneself may include having "a life" outside of the relationship with the person with BPD, the right to healthily assert oneself with the person with BPD, the right to define what one is willing to do and not do for the person with BPD, and the right to be guilt-free if living according to one's own values.

Reading and other resources for family/friends

Because of the limited time available in a short two-session intervention, the provision of a list of family/friends-focused reading to guide family/friends will be valuable and time efficient. You are most welcome to freely photocopy to give to family or friends where relevant the resources list below.

Books

The following books and one book chapter (alphabetical) were written primarily for families and friends of people with BPD or those in closely related circumstances. We have included our brief comments in brackets after the citation:

- Dobbs, B. (2008 Lulu.com). *When hope is not enough: a how-to guide for living with someone with borderline personality disorder.* (Written by a family member, as a deliberately concise easy read. Clearly articulates some core DBT concepts that are of great practical use. Compassionate and validating of the person with BPD and family members whilst simultaneously emphasizing how everyone can change and will benefit from change.)

- Fruzzetti, A. E. (2006). *Hi-conflict couple: a dialectical behaviour therapy guide to finding peace, intimacy and validation.* Oakland: New Harbinger. (This book draws from the "Family Connections" program for family/friends that the author codeveloped and expands on some DBT skills, especially validation. This book is suitable not only for "high-conflict" couples but also for all people wanting to improve the quality of their adult relationships.)

- Fruzzetti, A. E. (in press). *Families and borderline personality disorder: Lessening the pain—A dialectical behaviour therapy guide to finding peace and comfort in your family.* Oakland: New Harbinger (Based on Family Connections program concepts and skills.)

- Harvey, P. & Penzo, J. A. (2009). *Parenting a child who has intense emotions: dialectical behaviour therapy skills to help your child regulate emotional outbursts and aggressive behaviours.* Oakland: New Harbinger. (This book is intended for parents of children who are not yet adults drawing from DBT skills.)

- Kreger, R. (2008). *The essential family/friends guide to borderline personality disorder.* Center City: Hazelden. (This book tends to focus on people with BPD who have satisfactory or high self-esteem and view problems as lying externally to themselves and therefore do not frequently seek out mental health treatment, focusing less on those with poor self-esteem who do seek out treatment. Half the book is a practical how-to guide of skills that families can use.)

- Penney, D. & Woodward, P. (2005). Family perspectives on borderline personality disorder. Chapter 7. In: Gunderson, J. G. & Hoffman, P. D. (eds). *Understanding and treating borderline personality disorder: a guide for professionals and families.* Washington DC: American Psychiatric Publishing, 117–130. (Written by two family members who have been active prominent BPD advocates. Concise succinct chapter providing two brief family stories followed by guidance for family readers based on the authors' experiences.)

◆ Porr, V. (2010). *Overcoming borderline personality disorder: a family guide for healing and change.*Oxford: Oxford University Press. (Written by a family member who has been an energetic advocate for BPD research and treatment. The book covers all major aspects of BPD, including 140 pages of "tools" for family to use. The detail covered means that this 400-page book will also be suitable as a reference text.)

The following four books (alphabetical), which provide compassionate understandings of borderline personality disorder and its treatment, whilst written more for professionals and/or consumers, do have small sections specifically for families:

◆ Bockian, N. R., Porr, V., & Villagran, N. E. (2002). *New hope for people with borderline personality disorder.* New York: Three Rivers Press.

◆ Friedel, R. O. (2004). *Borderline personality disorder demystified: an essential guide for understanding and living with BPD.* New York: Marlowe.

◆ Gunderson, J. G. & Hoffman, P. D. (eds) (2005). *Understanding and treating borderline personality disorder: a guide for professionals and families.* Washington DC: American Psychiatric Publishing.

◆ Krawitz, R. & Jackson, W. (2008). *Borderline personality disorder: the facts.* Oxford: Oxford University Press. (Explicitly for consumers.)

National Education Alliance for BPD website

NEA-BPD is the largest international BPD advocacy organization, with family members and professionals on its extensive Board of Directors that includes most of the highly regarded and credible international BPD experts. For this reason, whilst we are usually cautious about recommending websites as they can change from providing accurate information that is helpful to providing inaccurate information that is not helpful, we do feel that we can recommend this site with reasonable confidence that it will continue to provide accurate and useful information for the foreseeable future.

The NEA-BPD website has a "Family/friends Guidelines" document (www. borderlinepersonality disorder.com—Families—Family/friends guidelines) that can be freely downloaded in A4 or booklet formats and printed to give to family/friends. Useful headings in the document include:

◆ Goals: go slowly
◆ Keep things cool and calm

- Maintain family routines
- Find time to talk
- Don't get defensive
- Self-destructive acts or threats require attention
- Listen
- When solving a family member's problems always involve the family member
- Develop strategies that everyone can stick to
- Limit setting
- Do not protect family members from the natural consequences of their actions
- Do not tolerate abusive treatment. Walk away and return to discuss the issue later
- Be cautious about using threats and ultimatums. They are a last resort (Gunderson & Berkowitz)

Friedel's website

Another website that we currently recommend is that of Robert Friedel (www.bpddemystified.com).

Friedel's website has a list of ten guidelines for families, partners, and friends that can be printed off and given to family/friends (Friedel). The headings of the ten guidelines are:

- Learn about the disorder
- Seek professional help
- Support the treatment program
- Respond consistently to problematic behaviors
- Attempt to remain calm
- Remain positive and optimistic
- Participate in educational experiences about borderline disorder
- Join a borderline disorder consumer and family support organization
- Remember the person with borderline disorder must take charge
- Take care of yourself

Multisession intervention

Multisession interventions might be anything from three sessions to 30 sessions and may take the form of any one of a number of formats depending on the unique circumstances of the person with BPD, their family/friends, and the resources available. These formats include couple sessions, family sessions involving client and family, and multifamily sessions with the person with BPD present or not present. Multisession interventions may involve support, education, psycho-education, skill enhancement (including communication, factual nonjudgmental descriptions, relationship effectiveness, problem solving, validation, empathy, and accurate expression of experience) or be more therapy focused, again depending on the unique circumstances of the person with BPD, their family/friends members, and the resources available.

A person with BPD who benefitted from a six-session multisession family intervention, illustrates the value of this work where resources are available:

> It is important for me to note how much my family and partner helped with my recovery and eventual wellness. Both my parents and husband found it extremely difficult in the beginning because like me, they didn't know anything about the condition. My mother and husband would attend sessions with Erica (therapist) occasionally, but my family really wanted to understand how to deal with me.
>
> There was a 6-week course held weekly in the evenings for families dealing with people with BPD. This course had a dramatic effect on me and my family. The group comprised parents mostly, plus a few brothers and sisters, trying to understand the people that they cared about. I think a lot of the people benefited from hearing the perspective of someone with the condition. I also found it rewarding trying to help people understand what it was like for the person with BPD and how they might be able to assist them.
>
> I listened to the families describing their experiences of living with someone with BPD. Hearing what it was like for people around me and the effect I was having on my family was another major turning point for me. I saw things for the first time through their eyes, realizing how preoccupied and self-absorbed I had been just trying to get through each day and cope with my own distress. This gave me perspective and a further opportunity to heal myself.
>
> I remember saying in one of the family group sessions though (and this is true)—a person with BPD is the only person who can really change things. Having support goes a long way to making the journey that bit easier, but unless someone is determined to put in the effort and hard work, all the help from family will not really make any difference. It has to come from within. Love, support, validation is all family and friends can do and I love my family and husband for all they have done to help me through. I am very lucky. My eyes still fill with tears when I read this last part. Tears of sadness for the difficult times I put them through and tears of joy for having come through it all, with their support.(Krawitz, 2008).

It will be valuable to know about multisession family options that are available whether provided by ourselves, our organization or outside individuals and organizations such as mental health family support groups (the latter are available in most cities). Clinicians interested in providing multisession family interventions formats are encouraged to seek out the related references.

The following reviews of working with couples and families might serve as a solid starting point

- Fruzzetti, A. E. & Iverson, K. M. (2006). Intervening with couples and families to treat emotion dysregulation and psychopathology. In: Snyder, D. K., Simpson, J. A., & Hughes, J. N. (2006) *Emotion regulation in couples and families: pathways to dysfunction and health.* Washington DC: American Psychological Association.

- Fruzzetti, A. E., Santisteban, D. A., & Hoffman, P. H. (2007). Dialectical behaviour therapy with families. In: Dimeff, L. A. & Koerner, K. (eds). *Dialectical behaviour therapy in clinical practice: applications across disorders and settings.*New York: Guilford, p. 222–244.

- Hoffman, P. D. & Fruzzetti, A, E, (2007). Advances in interventions with a relative with a personality disorder diagnosis. *Current Psychiatry Reports*9: 68–73.

- Porr, V. ((2010) Overcoming borderline personality disorder: a family guide for healing and change. Oxford: Oxford University Press.

Outcome research involving family/friends of people with BPD or BPD traits

STEPPS (Systems Training for Emotional Predictability and Problem-solving) is a 20-week skills-based community-based group program that often explicitly involves family/friends that is an add-on to existing BPD treatment. Significant people in the clients' community are invited to join the STEPPS program, with a view to assisting this community to effectively support and reinforce clients' movements towards effective behaviors. There are two randomized controlled trials of STEPPS effectiveness in two different centers, one in the USA and the other in Europe, and two further prepost studies demonstrating effectiveness (Black et al., 2008; Blum et al., 2008; Bos et al., 2010; Silk, 2008; van Wel et al., 2006).

Family Connections is a 12-session semistructured manualized (2 hours/ session) stand-alone community-based intervention for family/friends of people with BPD (those with BPD do not attend) run by family members and/or professionals. Family Connections was developed by Hoffman and Fruzzetti, and family members with the National Education Alliance for BPD, the largest international BPD advocacy organization, and continues to function under the auspices of this organization. Family Connections provides support, psychoeducation, and skills training based on DBT skills. Family Connections programs are run by trained family members or trained mental health professionals with an understanding, at least at the time of writing, that participants will not have to pay for the program themselves, apart from the cost of materials. Family Connections has been demonstrated in three prepost studies across three centers to be effective in reducing family/friends grief, depression, and burden, and improving perceptions of their relationships and experience of empowerment and mastery (Hoffman et al., 2005, 2007; Rajalin, et al., 2009). The geographic availability of Family Connections programs can be found by accessing the NEA-BPD website. A telephone adaptation of Family Connections has been recently developed for people living in areas where face-to-face Family Connections programs do not exist.

Family/friend comment

I found that the Family Connections program assisted me and others to feel more centered, empowered, and sure of ourselves. Generally, our loved ones with BPD started noticing these changes and that their family member was observing and sticking to limits. Over time this seemed to often result in the person with BPD finding a more centered place within themselves. And that was good news, indeed!

> ## Family/friend comment
>
> Since taking NEA-BPD's Family Connections course I feel more skilled at interacting with my daughter.

> ## Family/friend comment
>
> As a family member running Family Connections programs I am so proud of the Family Connections culture and tradition of volunteers leading the program. This generosity sets the stage for and gets the program off on the right footing. Participants experience this free or low-cost service as highly validating and welcoming, and in stark contrast to the many cool receptions we have previously been given.

Family members who are interested in attending a Family Connections program could be given the following Family Connections leader's description and perspective of the program.

> Penney, D. (2008). Family Connections: an education and skills training program for family member well being: a leader's perspective. *Social Work in Mental Health* 6: 229–241. Published simultaneously in Hoffman, P. D. & Steiner-Grossman, P. (eds). *Borderline personality disorder: meeting the challenges to successful treatment*. New York: Haworth Press 2008: 229–241.

DBT Family Skills Training (DBT-FST) is a 6–24-week multifamily program (2 hours/week) where BPD clients and their relatives attend and learn DBT-based skills with a particular emphasis on validation and accurate communication of experience (Hoffman, Fruzzetti, & Swenson, 1999). DBT-FST has been mentioned in Linehan's original 1993 DBT skills training manual (Linehan, 1993b, p. 37). DBT-FST demonstrated DBT clients and their relatives report high satisfaction with the intervention (Fruzzetti et al., 2007).

Multifamily DBT skills training: Multifamily DBT skills training has been part of an adaption for adolescents of standard adult DBT. The adaptation includes having family member/s attend the skills training groups along with their adolescent child. This adaptation was shown to be superior to treatment as usual for suicidal adolescents with BPD traits in a controlled trial (Rathus & Miller, 2002).

A **short series of family intervention sessions** have been shown in a case study series to have had a positive effect on the outcomes of people with severe BPD (Fruzzetti & Iverson, 2006).

MBT-A is an adaptation of MBT for adolescents with features of emerging personality disorder who self-harm and their families. A randomized controlled trial comparing MBT-A (family intervention with individual sessions for the adolescent) with treatment as usual demonstrated superior outcomes on a number of measures, including reduction in self-harm in the experimental group (Rossouw, in press).

I-BAFT is an intensive (3 sessions/week × 7 months) outpatient treatment model that integrates structural family therapy, DBT-informed individual therapy, and DBT skills training. Preliminary data on I-BAFT were promising in a case series of 13 adolescents with BPD (reported on in Fruzzetti et al., 2007).

McLean Hospital program

The McLean Hospital program (Gunderson, Berkowitz, & Ruiz-Sancho, 1997) adapted a program for families of people with BPD developed out of psychoeducational family interventions for schizophrenia. This program is without published data of effectiveness that we are aware of.

Outcome research of relevance to but not specific to family/friends of people with BPD

Validation skills taught to couples demonstrated that validating partner responses predicted stability and improvements in the affect of the other person in the couple (Fruzzetti & Iverson, 2006; Fruzzetti et al., 2007).

DBT skills for couples using a brief six-session group treatment demonstrated significant decreases in invalidation, increases in validation, decreased distress, and improved relationship satisfaction (Fruzzetti & Iverson, 2006; Fruzzetti et al., 2007).

A **DBT parenting skills intervention** with parents demonstrated decreased parent distress and their adolescent children (who did not attend the intervention) reported significantly decreased distress and psychopathology (Fruzzetti et al., 2007).

Appendix—Handout for family and friends

We have provided, as an appendix to this chapter, some information in the form of a brief handout for family and friends. You are most welcome to freely photocopy the appendix to give to family or friends where relevant.

BPD information

- One to six percent of people will meet diagnostic criteria for BPD sometime in their lives.
- Parents often report that they could tell something was wrong in the first year of their child's life.
- People with BPD have some brain differences to people without BPD (e.g., different sizes and functioning of some brain structures, sluggish serotonin system) [overactive "brain emotional petrol pedals" (amygdala) underactive "brain emotional brakes" (pre-frontal cortex) and sluggish "brain oil" (serotonin)].
- Experts agree that it is likely that biological and psychological factors are involved in causing BPD.
- Evidence of biological causal factors include five-fold increased rates of BPD in identical vs nonidentical twins where one twin has BPD; five-fold increased rate of self-harm where a particular gene is present.
- Evidence of psychological causal factors include higher rates of self-harm where childhood sexual abuse has occurred and higher rates of BPD where court-recognized childhood abuse has occurred.
- BPD can occur in caring families with neither the person with BPD nor parents to blame.
- Most people with BPD make substantial improvements over time such that they no longer have BPD.
- There are now a range of treatments demonstrated in gold standard research to be effective, including high-quality generalist treatment.
- A range of family and friend interventions have also been shown to be effective in moderately rigorous research.
- Higher family member involvement with the person with BPD has been shown in general (statistically) to be predictive of better outcomes for the person with BPD.
- Validation is when the other person knows that you "get it"—that is, know where they are coming from.

- Validation has been shown to be a highly effective action that family and friends can do, helping to improve the quality of relationships.
- We can all practice and improve our validation skills.
- Research shows that, in general, it is much more effective to reward someone (e.g., praise) after they do a behavior you like than to punish or criticize them after they do a behavior you do not like.
- Research shows that when rewarding someone, it is most effective to do so as soon as possible after the behavior that you like.
- We need to wait till the behavior that we want to encourage occurs and then reward the person as soon as possible thereafter.
- Sometimes the person with BPD does not like being praised (e.g., they feel pressure to perform), with praise actually inadvertently decreasing the likelihood of the behavior occurring again. In these situations, a reward other than praise will need to be found.
- Research shows that the lives of family members of people with BPD are challenging and difficult, with high levels of stress and burden experienced. We hope that as family and friends you will take excellent care of yourselves. All humans are deserving of compassion and the right to strive towards a happy life. If you are choosing to support a family member or friend with BPD, it is our belief also that the more content you are, the better you will be able to support the person with BPD.

Chapter 8

Top ten additional resource-efficient treatment strategies

Summary

- In this chapter we describe ten resource-efficient strategies that are additional to those previously described in the book.
- The ten strategies either have some direct evidence base in generalist mental health treatments or are drawn from effective evidence-based specialist BPD treatments.

Top ten strategies

1. Mentalizing and mindfulness
2. Valued action irrespective of emotions:
   a. including identification of emotion
   b. acceptance of emotions
3. Self-acceptance
4. Accepting thoughts and valued action
5. Changing thoughts
6. Decreasing hyperarousal
7. Chain analysis
8. Structure:
   a. joint crisis plans
   b. problem solving
   c. psychoeducation

9. Skills:

    a. DBT distress tolerance skills

    b. DBT interpersonal effectiveness skills

10. Clinical feedback of treatment outcomes[1]

In this chapter we describe ten strategies that are additional to those previously described in the book. The effective specialist BPD treatments that we have drawn mostly from in this chapter are DBT and mentalization-based therapy as these are the two BPD treatments with the most robust evidence base and they are the treatments with which we are most familiar (AB—mentalization-based therapy; RK—DBT).

The ten strategies either have some direct evidence base in generalist mental health treatments or are drawn from effective evidence-based specialist BPD treatments. In both these situations the evidence base for effectiveness of each individual strategy in BPD generalist mental health treatments is via proxy rather than a direct relationship. Nevertheless, we have included these strategies believing that they will be effective in BPD generalist mental health treatments and that they will assist the reader in a practical, clinical manner as they can be readily conceptualized and utilized by generalist mental health clinicians.

We are not suggesting that each technique will be immediately helpful to the patient but that the clinician can draw on the strategies during treatment of a person with BPD. To some extent the value that personality disordered individuals derive from treatment comes through experience of being involved in a carefully considered, well-structured, and coherent interpersonal endeavor. The techniques described here and throughout the book facilitate this. What may be helpful is the internalization of a thoughtfully developed structure, the understanding of the inter-relationship of different reliably identifiable components, the causal interdependence of specific ideas and actions, the constructive interactions of professionals, and above all the experience of being the subject of reliable, coherent, and rational thinking. These are all correlates of the level of seriousness and the degree of commitment with which clinicians and teams of professionals approach the problem of caring for people with

1. A modest amount of the content in this chapter has been adapted from Krawitz, R., Jackson, W. (2008). Borderline personality disorder: the facts. Oxford: Oxford University Press. The authors wish to thank Wendy Jackson and Oxford University Press for their permission to adapt and use the information from that book for consumers for this book for generalist mental health clinicians.

BPD. So in using the techniques described here the clinician is advised to do so within a carefully constructed framework in the generalist mental health setting.

1. Mentalizing and mindfulness

Mentalizing and mindfulness are terms used to describe, amongst other things, the self-reflective capacity to directly monitor our own thoughts, emotions, and actions. Mentalizing is the core hypothesized mechanism of change in mentalization-based therapy (Bateman & Fonagy, 1999, 2001, 2006, 2008a, 2009b) and is arguably a focus of attention for all effective psychological therapies (Allen et al., 2008). Mindfulness has stormed into western psychological practices with a growing evidence base (Roemer & Orsillo, 2008) and is a core part of DBT. Mentalizing and mindfulness constructs provide a broad "psychological mindedness" that involves being aware of thinking, emotions, and actions; being able to think about thinking, think about emotions and think about actions; and feeling about thinking, feeling about emotions, and feeling about actions, all changing not thoughts and emotions rather the person's relationship to their thoughts and emotions. There is an enhanced attention to and awareness of current experience or present reality characterized by "especially *open* or *receptive* awareness and attention" (Brown & Ryan, 2003).

Whilst the two concepts of mentalization and mindfulness differ in their scope, the practical use of them in generalist mental health settings overlaps, particularly in helping people become mindful of mind. The terms mentalizing and mindfulness signal a focus on mind rather than action. Explicated in Buddhism (Hahn, 1975), mindfulness was originally conceived as an enhanced attention to and awareness of current experience, requiring openness to sensation without judgment. Not restricted to any object or function, one can be mindful of a flower or of one's breathing or of others' behavior (Bateman, in press), but primarily we ask people to become mindful of their own mind, although this may become possible only through initially practicing being mindful of an external object or perhaps part of the body. Once someone is mindful of another mind and not just their own, they are mentalizing or involved in relationship mindfulness.

Patients are encouraged to be mindful of and mentalize all experiences both during and outside of the therapy session and during and after any significant experience. Mentalizing and being mindful of a recent past experience will be different from mentalizing and being mindful of an experience whilst it is happening. Mentalizing and being mindful of an experience after the experience has the advantage of being a slower process as the emotional intensity will have usually waned.

On the other hand, mentalizing and being mindful of current experience has the advantage of the experience and its details being immediately available to reflection. Being able to mentalize and be mindful of current experience is a challenging task but one that has the potential to change and revolutionize the lives of our patients. If our patients are able to both fully experience and reflect upon the experience as it is happening, known as mentalized affectivity (Jurist, 2005), they will have a vast amount of information available to them to assist effective decision-making in the moment. When our patients are able to string together a series of effective decisions they will be able to influence positively the course of their lives.

Mentalizing and mindfulness of current experience requires a rapidly shifting focus from full participation in the experience to a position of stepping back just enough to allow for some degree of self-observing and self-reflection, and then to throw oneself back into the experience and so forth. This gives a self-reflection loop inside the experience, enabling one to affect the outcome of the situation (Figure 8.1).

We need to be able to identify the need for stepping back, taking charge, stepping back, and being sure to not step back too far. If we step back too far we lose connection with the experience, resulting in an overly intellectual and unemotive position or even emotional numbness.

As clinicians we will be repeatedly encouraging client mentalizing and mindfulness by asking questions such as, "What are you thinking?", "What are you feeling?", "What do you make of this experience?" The goal is for patients to become expert at unraveling their experience, opening the experience up for

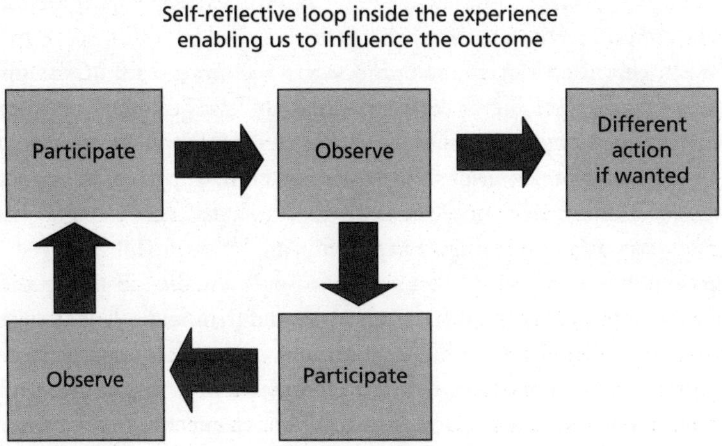

Fig. 8.1 Self-reflective loop inside the experience, enabling us to influence the outcome.

productive exploration. Mindfulness and mentalizing enable our patients to take ownership of their experiences, thereby influencing experience, including regulating actions and emotions.

Mentalizing and relationship-mindfulness also describe processes that include reflection on the world of other people in relation to the self which promotes empathy and reciprocity in relationships. Given that people with BPD are sensitive within interpersonal interactions it is important that the clinician focuses increasingly on mentalizing the relationship process, validating the patient's accurate experiences and responses, and exploring in detail possible misperceptions and disproportionate emotional responses.

Mindfulness and mentalizing are psychological skills requiring practice. Just like physical training gets muscles fit and enable us to carry out physical tasks we could not previously do, so is it with mindfulness and mentalizing. We need to encourage our patients to practice and train their minds to become fit and skilled at psychological skills, which are particularly relevant for our patients where emotional intensity often leads to automatic impulsive action.

Consumer comment

I used to consider mindfulness to be an "out there" eastern religious practice that was for people who looked and behaved differently to me. I thought that you had to sit silently and motionlessly for long periods of time. With this view, I could not see how it could possibly be part of my life.

I did not realize that mindfulness is just about paying attention—no more and no less, and that we all use mindfulness skills in our everyday life, for example paying attention to listening to our friends or paying attention to a mundane activity such as washing the dishes.

I took some mindfulness classes and, whilst like any other skill it required regular practice, was surprised at the simplicity. Mindfulness can be practiced anywhere, anytime, and for as long or as short as you choose, and can be an incredibly good way of settling intense emotions or letting time pass so the emotions settle themselves (Krawitz & Jackson, 2008).

The focus on mentalizing at the beginning of treatment annoyed me at first because it sounded like a stupid word. It was only when I realized that most of us fail to mentalize each other and that the problem was that my boyfriend had no idea what went on in my mind that I appreciated its importance. I asked my boyfriend to describe what he thought my feelings and ideas were about our relationship. He was completely wrong. I tried to do the same with him and it was really difficult. This helped us realize that we were always reacting to each other on silly assumptions that we thought were the truth. Not mentalizing was ruining our relationship. It was pretty simple to make it a bit better. All we had to do was to ask each other what was going on in our minds. Oddly this seemed very difficult at first but we became better at it as we paid more attention to it.

2. Valued action irrespective of emotions

Valued action

In addition to working with patients on changing thoughts and cultivating desired emotions, many, if not all, of the effective specialist BPD evidence-based treatments will encourage acceptance of primary emotions (see later) and valued action irrespective of unpleasant emotions, that is, we can take our emotions with us and still engage in effective skillful behavior.

Acceptance and commitment therapy is another mindfulness and acceptance-based behavior therapy that, like DBT, has taken its place in the psychological world with numerous publications and a growing evidence base of effectiveness (Powers, Zm Vorde Sive Vording, & Emmelkamp, 2009). In a nutshell, acceptance and commitment therapy encourages clients to accept their experience (including emotions) via mindfulness and to then engage in committed action in keeping with their own values. This construct, when shared with patients, can provide a simple framework on which to input information on emotions that encourages action outputs that are skillful and effective.

Values usually become apparent in discussion, but one can explore values with patients in a structured way using something like the motivational interviewing "values card sort" (freely available at www.motivationalinterview. org) or something like the exercises below.

From the following list, you might want to circle values that apply to you.

fun	money	friendship	family	integrity
energy	honesty	stimulation	structure	novelty
companionship	justice	creativity	compassion	success
humanity	caring	modern	traditional	autonomy
community	doing	being	change	acceptance
religion	spirituality	reliability	flexibility	firmness
fairness	kindness	artistic	organized	working
sport				

You may want to write down your five core (or central) values:

....

....

....

....

....

Fulfilment, meaning, and purpose

You might want to sit down quietly and brainstorm three or four things that you find fulfilling, meaningful or purposeful.

....

....

....

....

Consumer comment

I spent many years wondering who I was and what the meaning of my life was. I then discovered two areas in my life, especially, that I was and am good at and passionate about. I now put time and effort into these two areas.

One is my work. On enough days, I do make a small difference in someone's day. This gives me considerable pleasure and satisfaction. The other is my role to my nieces and nephew as "Aunty." I try to be the very best "Aunty" I can, and get a huge sense of satisfaction and self-worth from the effort I put into that role. After many years of searching for whom I was, I now feel I have a place in the world fulfilling these and other roles (Krawitz & Jackson, 2008).

Acceptance of emotions

Emotions just are

We teach patients that emotions are neither right nor wrong—they just are. Whether experiencing an emotion is helpful or harmful depends on how our patients act in response to the emotion. For example, it will be unhelpful if anger results in choosing to assault a person and ending up in prison but helpful and effective if anger leads to avoiding people who are unsafe. Sexual feelings can be harmful if they lead to unsafe sex or helpful if they lead to pleasure. Feelings of wanting human connection can harmfully lead to getting together with people who use or abuse or can lead to making satisfying relationships.

Emotions have important functions

As our patients have often had devastating lives and experiences, it is understandable that they more commonly than not view emotions, especially displeasing emotions, as something negative to be got rid of. Emotions take their mind "off line" (Arnsten, 1998), they cannot think, and unleash panic. This leads to emotion avoidance by actions such as self-harm, substance use, dissociation, bulimia, and leading a restricted life. This understandable approach, while effective in the short term at decreasing distress, serves only to reinforce the notion that emotions, and especially displeasing emotions, are dangerous and to be avoided, thereby preventing learning skills required to live an active fulfilling life.

To counter this we teach patients that emotions can be useful gauges and have important functions. When we are presented with a situation, our brains quickly evaluate the situation, comparing it to past experience and reacting with an emotion. Emotions provide information about ourselves and our environment, and are essential for effective decision-making and action. Fear and anger can warn us of impending danger and cause us to move or avoid a situation, sadness can tell us that what we are sad about is something of value to us and happiness encourages us to recreate the situation resulting in happiness.

So, the goal is for therapist and client to explore how our patients may find a way to begin to experience emotions early on when the emotions are small and not overwhelming, and when they can have a decent chance at using the information from their emotions to generate effective functioning, including the cultivation of desired emotions. Being alert to early warnings in the mind or body is done through maintaining mentalizing and being mindful of mind. We do reassure patients that keeping emotions away, such as by choosing to distract themselves, can remain an effective skill to have in reserve, provided they use this sparingly and consciously. It is important, however, that our patients do this as little as possible so that they can learn that emotions are not to be feared and they can gradually begin to access the benefits of awareness of their emotions.

Commitment to and practice of awareness of emotions can significantly contribute to client recovery. Patients can practice by taking a moment, a minute or five minutes once or several times a day to reflect on what they are feeling and putting a name to that emotion. The first steps in this process are identification and acceptance, preferably welcoming acceptance, of all emotion, including distressing emotions.

Identification of emotions

As examples of psychoeducation on emotions we describe how we teach patients to identify four emotions: anger, fear, sadness, and happiness.

Anger

We teach that anger is a stress response to real or perceived danger and causes a rush of adrenalin and increased blood flow to muscles. Muscles may tense up, especially in the shoulders and neck, as the body gets ready to fight or run (fight/flight response). We might be aware of clenched teeth, fist-making or folded arms. Our heart and breathing may speed up and we may be thinking critical thoughts.

Fear

We teach that fear is also a stress response to real or perceived danger and also causes a rush of adrenalin, and we may experience some of the same body responses as with anger (tight muscles, rapid breathing). There may be an experience of dread and anxiety, and an urge to get away. Thoughts may be worry type of thoughts.

Sadness

We teach that sadness often occurs in response to a loss (recent or past) of something we value or valued. Sadness may be felt physically as a lump in the throat, a sense of heaviness or a sense of emptiness. Energy may be low. Many people cry when they are sad. Thoughts may be negative, pessimistic or focused on particular sad events.

Happiness

We teach that happiness is more likely to occur when we are engaged in activities that are pleasurable, purposeful or meaningful, and when we are relaxed or remembering a positive experience. Happiness may be experienced as a sense of lightness, contentment or fulfillment. We may be energetic, having a "spring in our step." We may feel peaceful and at one with the world. We may feel buoyant and confident. Thoughts may be positive, optimistic, and hopeful.

Riding the wave

We share with you "Riding the Wave," written by colleagues of ours for one of their treatment groups.

Riding the Wave

One way of thinking about our emotions is to think of them like the ocean. If you imagine the sea, you might picture it as flat, calm and blue, or as crashing surf, or small rocking waves.

Just as the ocean can change, so can emotions. With the ocean, it is the weather that might cause changes—high winds or still sunny days can make a difference to how the waves react. In our lives, it can be problems with friends or family, stress about school, things that happen in our environment and around us that may affect our emotions.

Sometimes you can see a storm brewing that might whip the waves up, other times the change may happen with little warning. But what we know for certain, about the sea and about our emotions—they chop and change.

So, like waves, our emotions may at one moment be calm and serene, and at another rocky and angry. We might float along on a happy emotion, or be swept away by anger, we might experience small emotional ups and downs, or we might get dumped by a big wave of sadness and hopelessness.

We can either let our emotions push us around and move us along—or we can learn how to harness our emotions. We can learn to float with our feelings, letting them wash over us, or how to surf the big feelings, not letting them crash over us, but taking control, and riding the wave!

This group is about learning how to ride the waves of emotion—not to be swept away by them, but to recognize weather changes (emotional warning signs), go with the flow, and deal with getting wet. Once you know how to ride the waves, you should have the skills with you to surf any breaker that comes your way.

Kindly printed with the permission of Kari Centre Riding the Wave DBT Program

Consumer comment

I never used to let my angry feelings out, except by turning it upon myself. I was scared that if I started to let it out it would never stop. This assumption proved to be untrue. Now I attempt to deal with anger as it arises, trying to learn what my feelings are telling me and looking for ways to address the situation I am in (Krawitz & Jackson, 2008).

Primary and secondary emotions

A primary emotion is an emotion that is experienced in response to an event. A secondary emotion is an emotion about the primary emotion on the basis of beliefs, usually self-critical beliefs, about the primary emotion. Other writers conceptualize emotions as basic and social in nature, taking a more biological and adaptive approach (Panksepp, 1998). This differentiation, along with the distinction between primary and secondary emotion, is discussed in more detail in the section on tolerance of primary and secondary emotions in Chapter 4. In SCM this distinction is made and is discussed with patients along with the division of emotions into primary and secondary emotions.

As a reminder, suffice it to say that to be less distressed by their emotions, patients need to be more welcoming and accepting of their primary or basic emotions whatever they are. This includes not only emotions that are pleasurable but also those that are distressing, including sadness, anxiety, and anger. If patients are able to do this, and act skillfully whatever their primary emotion, then they are left with their primary emotion only, without the additional burden of the secondary emotions. This can lift a great weight from their shoulders and their lives.

Distress happens—valued action we can choose

Extreme distress can result in our patients choosing behaviors designed to decrease the pain and distress in the short term that end up making things even worse, that is, mood-dependent actions. Emotions themselves, even distressing emotions, are not necessarily a problem. Our task is to act skillfully and effectively in accordance with our personal values despite distressing feelings or moods; that is, to take non-mood-dependent actions.

Consumer comment

I tried avoiding feeling a lot of the time. When I then felt something like being angry, sad or happy, I would give myself a hard time and feel guilty for feeling what I did. This made every emotion more distressing. Once I learned to be fully present in the moment, and accept how I felt, I was able to work on managing the primary emotion, and thereby gain some control of my emotional states (Krawitz & Jackson, 2008).

3. Self-acceptance

Acceptance is a core construct and explicit skill taught and practiced in DBT, is implicit in parts of the effective evidence-based specialist BPD psychodynamic therapies, and has been central to Buddhist psychological practices for thousands of years.

Standard approaches for addressing low self-esteem might include naming or inviting our patients to look for or build attributes, qualities, skills or achievements, with therapist and client reinforcing all the above behaviors. However, these standard interventions that often work for less self-loathing patients are frequently experienced by severe chronic self-loathing patients with BPD as discordant with their self-loathing perception. This may result in therapists' well-meaning efforts to increase client self-worth to actually be experienced by patients as invalidating and therefore damaging of the therapeutic alliance or trigger a deepening of patients' self-loathing, setting back the client's journey towards positive self-worth. It is essential that clinicians recognize this. The use of standard, rationally determined interventions, such as weighing up evidence for a belief, is a common way to create iatrogenic interactions with people with BPD. In mentalization-based treatment this is conceived as failing to recognize that the patient's experience is held in psychic equivalence—in this state of mind a thought is a fact and has no "as if" quality and as such cannot be argued against. To do so, as we mentioned, merely invalidates the patient's experience and makes them feel misunderstood.

In these situations a goal of a single moment of acceptance might interrupt the vicious locked-in downward self-generating spiral of self-loathing. Patients might validate how understandable it was that they got to the present situation of self-loathing, for example "It makes perfect sense that I am so self-critical currently given my past", "It is sad that I currently feel fundamentally flawed, however this makes sense given … " (Huber, 2001). Instead of self-invalidating with, "I am bad, rotten, and despicable" our patients might self-validate by saying, "Given my childhood experiences of being told that I was bad, rotten, and despicable, it is no wonder that I feel bad, rotten, and despicable and have yet to feel good about myself." This can have the effect of shifting stuck self-loathing to fluid sadness, anger, and grieving.

Dysfunctional unhelpful self-criticism of any single event can serve as a stimulus for patients to consider choosing self-acceptance instead. DBT languages this choosing of acceptance as "turning the mind," deliberately using metaphorical language of action (turning) that emphasizes that acceptance is a deliberate choice that one can make (Linehan, 1993b). The pathway to self-acceptance is almost always a journey of small steps, with each nonself-acceptance moment or event being an opportunity to "turn the mind" to increased self-acceptance and each moment of self-acceptance being an opportunity to celebrate.

Huber, Zen teacher, uses koans that invite self-acceptance by starting with self-acceptance of this moment of self-criticism or nonself-acceptance, "If I could have compassion for hating myself, I would no longer be hating myself, I'd be loving myself, and nothing about me would need to change." Koans serve the purpose of surprise, intending to help our patients break out of automatic stuck positions. Koans need to avoid being seen to be gimmicky and must be used by the therapist from a place of compassion and warmth, with the therapist ready to back off or apologize when the intervention misses the mark. Patients may put a floor under their self-generating spiral of self-loathing by naming that they are not very good at self-accepting *yet* (Zelan, on DBT-Listserv, 2010).

Research is increasingly showing that whilst self-esteem and self-compassion are both related to psychological health, self-compassion is more positively correlated to psychological health than self-esteem (Neff, 2009). Neff (2009) provides a definition of self-esteem based on the work of William James (1890), "The degree to which the self is judged to be competent in life domains deemed important," and includes that self-esteem is also usually linked with what others think of one (social rank). As self-esteem is based on day-to-day achievements that determine self-worth, it has been shown to be less stable than self-compassion as a determinant of self-worth (Neff & Vonk, 2009). Self-esteem is felt when things are going well, whereas self-compassion and self-acceptance can be at their strongest when most needed, when things are not going well. Self-compassion and self-acceptance can then be psychologically effective in dealing with rough times and shame in a way that self-esteem cannot. Self-acceptance also does not require that the person change their evaluation of themselves, "only" that the person accepts the common humanity of failings. As self-acceptance is not contingent upon a positive view of oneself, it can occur alongside feelings of inadequacy (Neff, 2009) and so might be a more useful earlier intervention with patients who are severely self-loathing. Similarly, Neff (2009) proposes that as self-compassion is more stable and not contingent on external sources, it may be a more useful pathway to psychological health than self-esteem and may be easier for some self-loathing patients than increasing self-esteem.

Client self-acceptance is to be balanced with patients changing things about themselves that they wish to change. It is actually very self-compassionate to work towards becoming whom we aspire to be in the future. In this way self-compassion is not synonymous with passivity and stagnation; in fact often quite the opposite.

Consumer comment

I was, and still am to some extent, very hard on myself—I expected nothing less than perfection, and anything a fraction short of perfection was a failure—another of my many failures. Over time I have learnt that like every other human, there are some things I am better at than others, and I was not going to be perfect at everything I did and every interaction I had with someone. Learning to accept that I am OK, even if I am not perfect, has been a big learning curve with great rewards. I am much more casual now about minor things, "not sweating the small stuff." With important activities, whilst I still strive to do my very best, I am much more accepting if things don't work out. After all, how could I ask myself to do any more than my best? I am much kinder now towards myself, which helps me go about my world with a lightness I never had before (Krawitz & Jackson, 2008).

---

4. Accepting thoughts and valued action

DBT and other acceptance-based behavior therapies will often invite patients to mindfully note and accept their thoughts as a major intervention in and of itself. Mentalization-based therapy also encourages patients to accept their thoughts as a starting point for mentalizing or mind-exploring, and emphasizes the process of thinking and experiencing more than the content. To this extent the clinician is always reminded that the focus in the majority of the ten resource-efficient strategies described in this chapter is often more on changing the *relationship* of the person *to* their thoughts and feelings than it is trying to help them *change* the thoughts and feelings themselves.

DBT and other mindfulness and acceptance-based behavior therapies encourage patients to note and accept (sometimes using a golf clicker as a monitoring tool) self-critical thoughts as a means of what acceptance and commitment therapy refers to as "de-fusion"; not backing away from the truth as the person sees it, but separating fact from thought. That is, a thought is just a thought and what the person is thinking may be a fact, but may not be a fact. This might take the form of, "I am noticing a thought of self-loathing." This approach of looking at the process of thinking more than the content of thinking might be more acceptable to patients with severe self-loathing who might view efforts at cognitive modification as further proof of the fundamentally flawed nature of their thinking and therefore their entire selves. Therapists will then encourage skillful committed valued action that is not dependent on positive self-esteem thoughts. That is, patients need to take their thoughts with them as they engage in valued action. This is the cognitive equivalent of nonmood-dependent behavior. We all need to act skillfully in the direction of our life goals, whatever our mood and thoughts are. When as therapists we are not explicitly inviting patients to accept their thoughts, we can still seamlessly respond to patients self-critical statements with a defusion comment. For example, in response to patients saying, "I am bad and rotten," as therapists we can seamlessly say, "and now you are having the thought that you are bad and rotten."

5. Changing thoughts

Cognitive modification has been well demonstrated to be highly effective in the treatment of a range of mental health conditions, especially anxiety and depressive disorders (Wright et al., 2006), and is part of DBT. For your ease of recall and use we share the acronym JACOB (adapted from Auckland SAFE group), which we and our patients have found helpful. Below is a psychoeducation handout on the acronym that you are most welcome to freely photocopy and give to your patients where relevant. All the components of JACOB are indicators of nonmentalizing.

JACOB (adapted from Auckland SAFE group)

- **J**umping to conclusions
- **A**ttributing personally
- **C**atastrophizing
- **O**vergeneralizing
- **B**lack and white thinking

Jumping to conclusions

This type of thought pattern occurs when we don't wait to hear a full explanation or to get enough information to make an accurate assessment of a situation. We *jump to a conclusion* without sufficient evidence. We can challenge this by stopping and taking a breath before we panic or overreact and think to ourselves, "Do I have all the information I need?" and "What other information do I need before I can make a wise evaluation of the meaning?" Mind reading is a form of *jumping to conclusions*. Have you ever been asked to attend a meeting and immediately thought, "What have I done wrong?" This is an example of *jumping to a conclusion* without the information we need to develop an informed opinion. The person inviting us may be wishing to congratulate us, seek out our valuable opinion or discuss a pay rise with us and our angst will have been fruitless. When somebody yawns, we might *jump to a conclusion* that they find us boring, when in fact they may be sleep deprived, have had a long hard day or be someone that yawns a lot whoever they are with.

Attributing personally

Attributing personally refers to an automatic assumption that a negative event or experience is our fault without evidence for this. We may excessively personalize things, attributing a disproportionate amount of responsibility to ourselves. For example, "I am useless at keeping friends, if only I had made more of a special effort, my friend would not have moved town." We need to ask ourselves, "How much of what is happening is about ourselves, other people or the situation?"

Catastrophizing

Most of us have been in a situation where we are meeting someone and the other person is delayed. Do we immediately presume we have been stood up because they do not like us, or that they have been involved in a dreadful motor vehicle accident, or do we entertain the possibility that they may have had a flat tire or the babysitter was late? Catastrophizing occurs when we assume the worst possible outcome from a situation without giving thought or weight to other possible outcomes. This is the opposite of hopefulness, where we look "for a favourable outcome within the realm of possibilities" (Clarke, 2003). Decreasing *catastrophic thinking* and increasing hopefulness is important because we are more likely to feel better whilst being realistically hopeful. Being hopeful has been shown to improve our energy to take action that then results in greater likelihood of achieving our goals. If we are *catastrophizing*, we will also have a belief that what has happened or will happen will be unbearable and that, "I will not be able to stand it." We can challenge *catastrophic thinking* and invite realistic hopefulness by asking ourselves, "Am I thinking the worst?", "What is the likelihood or probability of this occurring?", "Could I survive if that outcome occurred?" or where appropriate saying to ourselves, "If the worst happens, I will not like it, however, I will be able to stand it."

Overgeneralizing

This occurs when in response to a single negative event we generalize this excessively (*overgeneralize*) to all areas of our lives. For example, after a setback we might say, "See, I am useless at everything." We may overestimate the degree to which future negative events will take place on the basis of a current negative event. There is a filtering of the event so that we focus on negatives whilst discounting or being unaware of positives. Do our language, thoughts, and self-talk frequently contain words like "all," "every," "no one," "never," "everybody," or "nobody?" These words often indicate that we are *overgeneralizing* as it is very uncommon, for example, that, "good things *never* happen," "*all* men are ... ," or "*all* women are ... ". Changing these words to "frequently," "sometimes," "maybe" or "occasionally" can help us to live in the world with greater lightness.

Black-and-white thinking

Alternative ways that you may have heard *black-and-white thinking* described are *all-or-nothing, absolutist or dichotomous thinking*. When we engage in *black-or-white thinking*, we only see two options. Often these two options are *all-good* or *all-bad* and often they involve judgments about ourselves and others. The people we like probably have some features that we do not like that much, and people we dislike will probably have some redeeming features. *Black-and-white thinking* often involves us being harshly critical of ourselves. This harsh self-judgment will keep our energy for change low. It is hard for anyone to get motivated when they are being told off and scolded. Try changing, for example, "I am useless at everything" to "I can ... " (e.g., cook, run a home, listen well), and "Nobody ever does anything for me" to "Jill rang me, John listened to me."

When evaluating a situation we may only see two choices—the *absolute* right choice and the *absolute* wrong choice, when in reality most choices have advantages and disadvantages. We might believe that there is only one right way to do things. In actual fact there are hundreds of shades between black and white, and often there are many solutions or ways of looking at a situation.

How many ways do you think there are to make an omelet? We can think of about six ways, all probably likely to turn out a good tasty omelet, even if the method was not the one we previously would have seen as the right way. Also, if we cooked six omelets in different ways and gave them to 100 readers, I am sure we would see a wide range of people's preferences—thank goodness!

We need to try avoiding the *all-or-nothing* route. If we can't clean our house from top to bottom, including the ceilings and every window, it can still be worthwhile washing the dishes or tidying up the lounge. When our patients see the range of possibilities in situations, you will know that they have taken a giant step in their recovery—they will be mentalizing again. It takes practice to look for the range of possibilities and options.

Self-loathing

Inviting clients to consider whether they were born self-loathing can sometimes be a cognitive strategy to invite patients to open to the idea that instead of feeling they were born with "original sin" or fundamentally flawed, to consider whether people (including themselves) might have been born with "original self-acceptance" or "original self-neutrality." We have found the simple statement "we all have an equal right to be on this planet, and an equal right to strive for contentment" to be well accepted cognitively by most clients. Whilst it is another thing to emotionally accept this statement, the cognitive acceptance provides a useful starting point with some traction.

Exploration of fallibility as a normative part of the human condition ("everyone makes mistakes") can be a useful change-based cognitive strategy whilst simultaneously validating patients' and our common human fallibility (Gilbert, 2009, 2010; Neff & Vonk, 2009). Patients can be encouraged to consider the common humanity of problems and failures, "problems and failures do not define me—everyone has problems and failures." Some clients will experience the cognition that they are not alone in their suffering as invalidating of the uniqueness of their situation, whilst others might find this validating and encouraging of self-compassion. "How would you relate to someone else with your unique circumstances?" might be a useful cognitive strategy for those who are more compassionate and empathic to others than to themselves.

6. Decreasing hyperarousal

Mentalization-based therapy and DBT both emphasize the importance of optimal client emotional arousal that will promote mentalizing and skillful behavior.

A stable secure attached therapy relationship promotes optimal emotional arousal and in turn mentalizing. Mentalizing promotes optimal arousal and an optimal therapy relationship. Therapist and patient validation of patients' intense emotional experience supports patients lessening their emotional hyperarousal. Patients can be encouraged to directly decrease their emotional hyperarousal using a range of mentalization, mindfulness, self-validation, distress tolerance, and emotion regulation skills. This will include encouraging self-compassionate behaviors where the person looks after or cares for themselves in the short and long term.

Intense emotions may compromise cognitive processing to such a degree that many skills shown to be effective in less severe emotion dysregulation that require higher cognitive processing such as standard cognitive-behavioral problem-solving can be impossible and what is required are distraction skills, especially those directly targeting physiological arousal (relaxation, temperature change, strenuous exercise) provided these are not medically contraindicated (Linehan, Bohus, & Lynch, 2007).

Discussing the need to decrease emotional hyperarousal in a biological or evolutionary context may be experienced as more acceptable and perhaps even validating for severe self-loathing clients. Gilbert describes how one can validate clients' hyperarousal from an evolution perspective (Gilbert, 2009, 2010), that is, those of our ancestors that were easily aroused to threat (including false positives of hyperarousal to threats that did not exist) were those that survived. Validation in a biological context can be described as the need to reduce stimulation of an overactive amygdala so that one can calm down, get new information in, and thus be able to make better choices (Long on DBT-Listserv, 2010). Gilbert (2010) brings together evolutionary and biological contexts proposing that self-compassion decreases emotional hyperarousal by deactivating the threat system (perhaps via stimulating oxytocin release) and by feelings of connection with others who might be suffering. Gilbert suggests that in this way hyperarousal, lack of safety, and insecure attachment feelings can be countered.

Where clients are dismissive or disdainful of terms such as self-compassion, self-acceptance or self-soothing, they may be more receptive to the language of "self-calming" because it is effective rather than being kind to or accepting of oneself (Long on DBT-Listserv, 2010), which might be a bridge too far where severe self-loathing exists.

7. Chain analysis

One way of clients monitoring themselves and the world around them is via a formal or informal chain analysis (Figure 8.2), with the term "chain" being used as a metaphor for the joined links that result in an end behavior. We will use the term "chain analysis," which has the same meaning as "functional analysis," "behavioral analysis," "problem and solution analysis," and mentalizing functional analysis. Formal explicit chain analyses are a central component of cognitive-behavioral therapy, whose evidence base for an extensive range of mental health conditions, including depression and anxiety disorders, has been well established (Wright et al., 2006), is central to DBT practice, and is explicit and implicit in mentalization-based therapy ("So how did you get from that to this?", "Let's stop and rewind what happened").

A chain analysis outlines the chain of internal and external events and links that led up to and came after a problem behavior (and sometimes solution behavior). The chain analysis or mentalizing analysis in MBT includes identification of the chain of mental states that led up to the behavior and those that followed. MBT and DBT places equal or usually greater focus on the mental aspect of the process as on the events themselves, emphasizing the mental processes that the patient needs to become "mindful" of, if they are to avoid problem behaviors. This is more than undertaking a chain analysis of a thought or emotion. It is more akin to actively focusing on how thoughts and emotions are held and identifying their quality. For example, someone may have a thought and react primarily to the content rather than reflect on the rigidity with which the thought is held. The latter may be the most important aspect and tracing the move from a flexible thought to a rigid thought may hold the key to change. The aim here is to engage the client in reflection to help them attend to a wider range of mental information to draw upon as they nuance and manage their emotions, thoughts, and actions. The aim of the chain analysis is to identify problems in the chain of events that occurred and then to explore solutions that will better prepare clients the next time they are in a similar position. Other therapies utilize this process in one way or another. In cognitive behavioral therapy chain analyses will be formal, often written down, and will be a central component of treatment. Other therapies will also be interested in the sequence of internal and external events that led to problems or successful solutions.

From the range of cognitive behavioral language for chain analyses we have chosen to use DBT language, as DBT is the dominant BPD cognitive behavioral treatment. We wish to acknowledge Linehan and Behavioural Tech for the terms "chain analysis," "problem analysis," "solution analysis," "vulnerability factors," "prompting event," "links," "problem behavior," "consequences," and "repair," and for the ideas (along with other cognitive behavioral clinicians) on which this section on chain analysis is based.

> Vulnerability factors ⇒ Prompting event ⇒ Links
> (thoughts, emotions, actions, and external events)
> ⇒ Problem behavior ⇒ Consequences ⇒ Repair

Fig. 8.2 Chain analysis. Reproduced from Krawitz, R. and Jackson, W. *Borderline Personality Disorder*, p.154 © Oxford University Press, 2008, with permission.

Problem behavior

Problem behavior is anything client and therapist define as a problem—it may be self-harm, using substances, yelling at children, assault, gambling, unsafe sex, numbing out, dissociating, binge eating or deliberate vomiting. Urges to problematic behaviors can also be the subject of chain analysis, for example urges to suicide, self-harm, use substances, gamble, leave therapy, etc. Emotions and thoughts can also be the subject of chain analysis (e.g., sadness or anxiety). We encourage being specific about exactly what the problem behavior was and when it happened. Starting a formal chain analysis with the problem behavior keeps us focused on the purpose of the chain analysis, which is to identify problems and solutions. Defining urges as targets of intervention encourages awareness of links in the chain of events when it is still possible for clients to reflect and do something differently. It also reminds the clinician and client to focus on mental process rather than solely on a series of external events or things that happened. For example, early warning signs of urges to leave therapy can prevent automatic impulsive leaving of therapy; early warning signs of numbing out can result in preventing further dissociation.

Vulnerability factors

Explore with your client the events that made your client vulnerable or predisposed to the problem behavior. Vulnerability factors are temporary factors that leave us susceptible to problem behaviors. For example, was your client tired, sleep deprived, physically unwell, premenstrual, having money worries or arguing with a shop assistant? As you and your client do more chain analyses you and they will begin to see patterns, and can then look at trying to reduce vulnerability factors where this is possible. For example, tending to painful medical and dental conditions will maximize health and decrease pain, leaving patients more resilient to face the challenges that life throws at them and more resilient in the face of prompting events. In the same way improving sleep will result in patients being more refreshed and resilient to face the challenges and to enjoy the pleasures of the day.

Prompting event

Look hard for what pushed your client's buttons to start the process of thoughts, emotions, and actions that led to the problem behavior. Once a pattern of prompting events is identified, a decision can be made whether it will be wise or unwise to avoid this particular prompting event in the future. Sometimes it will be wise to avoid the prompting event. Avoiding being near alcohol, wherever possible, is wise for almost all people who are early in their recovery from alcohol problems. On other occasions it will be impossible to avoid the prompting event. Such an example might be when night-time is a prompting event. For other events, patients will wisely and deliberately choose not to avoid the prompting event so that they can practice and get better skilled in the face of it. This will leave patients more resilient as life, of course, is full of potential triggering events. An example might be being cued/triggered by interaction with men. Often we cannot control prompting events occurring but our patients can learn to plan solutions for when the prompting event occurs. Of course, once our patients become skilled at dealing with previously triggering events the events will cease triggering them.

Links (thoughts, emotions, actions, and external events)

Thoughts, emotions, and actions interact with one another, which can lead to more thoughts, emotions, and actions, accentuating the distress leading to the problem behavior. Solutions may include putting in place more effective ways of thinking and acting that will lead to skillful actions in future to break the chain. Solution planning is the development of a "toolbox" of skills to allow patients to embrace alternative healthier actions.

Consequences

Often the consequences of problem behavior can become a new prompting event, creating a deteriorating downward spiral. Recognizing and naming consequences can be a good start to breaking this cycle.

Repair

Patients' problem behaviors may have a negative impact not only upon themselves but also on others. If this is the case, patients might wish to consider making a repair or some way to make amends.

Figure 8.3 is based on ideas of Marsha M. Linehan, LLC, Behavioural Tech, and Seth Axelrod. You and your client might want to write problems and solutions in different colors. Alternative ways of doing the chain analysis is to write the thoughts, emotions, and actions down on a piece of paper and join them with linking arrows.

Hurdles

If patients have not done this type of thing before, it will be unfamiliar and can be very challenging. By their very nature, chain analyses are usually designed to highlight problems that patients have had. This can be very hard. None of us particularly like our faults being scrutinized and known to others. So, be gentle and compassionate with your patients as they engage in this courageous and honest exploration. We can also partially balance the difficulties of doing

Vulnerability factors	Problem analysis	Solution analysis
Prompting event		
Links (thoughts, emotions, actions, and external events)		
Problem behavior		
Consequences for self		
For others		
Repair		

This figure is based on ideas of Marsha M Linehan, Behavioural Tech LLC, and Seth Axelrod.

Fig. 8.3 Chain analysis. Reproduced from Krawitz, R. and Jackson, W. *Borderline Personality Disorder*, p.154 © Oxford University Press, 2008, with permission.

a chain analysis by validating whatever we can in the chain that the client did skillfully or that at least made sense to us. Doing chain analyses of successful skillful behaviors can provide a balance if the going gets too tough just doing chain analyses of problem behaviors. The rewards of chain analyses may not be immediately apparent, but the rewards of persisting can be considerable. With practice the process can become second nature and skilled patients can find themselves using naturally and informally in their everyday lives, becoming a very effective recovery tool for the rest of their lives.

Consumer comment

I used to firmly believe that my impulsive actions "just happened." Learning to slow the process down enabled me to put in place solutions and avert or minimize unwanted action. This gave me choices, a sense of power and helped me maintain healthier friendships (Krawitz & Jackson, 2008).

Consumer comment

I really disliked chain analyses when I was first introduced to them. It was not easy for me to publicly explore my problems in exquisite detail. I found chain analyses frequently unpleasant as they often led to distressing emotions. I did them reluctantly because it was expected of me, and if ever I could get out of doing one I did. However, despite my initial reluctance I did lots, and began to discover that my chain of thoughts, emotions, and actions often followed similar patterns with similar outcomes. I began to recognize these patterns and started identifying parts of the patterns earlier on in the chain when they reoccurred. In time I learned healthier solutions which I would practice so that I could put these into action when I identified going down familiar pathways (Krawitz & Jackson, 2008).

8. Structure

Joint crisis plans

A single randomized controlled trial showed that crisis plans were promisingly effective in the treatment of people with psychosis or nonpsychotic bipolar disorder (Henderson et al., 2004, 2009; Flood et al., 2006). In the area of BPD, patients in the SCM vs mentalization-based therapy study rated crisis plans as *the* most important part of their treatment from a range of options related to individual and group therapy (Bateman & Fonagy, 2009b). This was true for patients in both groups and was rated just above "attention of my therapist to my goals" and "taking my experiences seriously." A randomized controlled trial is currently underway assessing the use of joint crisis plans in the treatment of people with BPD (Moran et al., 2010).

A joint crisis plan is collaboratively drawn up by patients and clinicians at a time of calm to plan ahead for future crises. The plan will be available to guide patients when they are in a crisis and likely to be sufficiently emotionally distressed that skillful actions that were easy enough to think about ahead of time cannot be accessed. The plan basically reminds patients about solutions that they themselves have come up with before. The plan also outlines what can and cannot be provided and who is responsible for what. It might well be that the process of discussing and negotiating the development of a crisis plan is as important as the actual content (Bateman & Fonagy, 2009a). The plan also will be available to crisis workers, guiding them as to the specifics of what clients will find useful.

Consumer comment

I never wanted to prepare for crises—surely every crisis would be the last. It was hard for me to accept that learning to manage crises was an important part of my recovery—to me that was like accepting that crises were OK. And guess what?—I now know that difficult times happen to all of us and what we all require is to simply know how to get through the difficult times. Although reluctant, I was persuaded to develop a written plan to deal with crises, which sat in my drawer unused for a very long time. One day, in yet another crisis, I decided I wanted to do something differently—I was totally sick of the crisis routine—so I looked at the plan and did some things in it—with some success. Whilst it took some while for the frequency and intensity of crises to reliably decrease, by accepting crises would occur and having strategies to manage them, I eventually learnt to deal with distressing times better (Krawitz & Jackson, 2008).

Problem-solving

Cognitive behavioral therapies, including the specialist BPD treatments DBT and STEPPS, and SCM, all provide problem-solving psychoeducation and practice to patients. This psychoeducation and practice provides a simple structure for problem-solving roughly as follows:

◆ Identify the problem (be as specific as possible).
◆ Brainstorm a range of solutions.
◆ Pick the most likely solutions.
◆ List the advantages and disadvantages of each solution.
◆ Pick the best solution.
◆ Develop an action plan (this can include accepting the situation and choosing to do nothing).
◆ Troubleshoot (this may include role-rehearsal).
◆ Take action.
◆ Evaluate the outcome.
◆ Review and adapt as required.

While this may seem obvious, it is often not the case for many of our patients, who often find the structure both novel and guiding.

Psychoeducation

A brief psychoeducation workshop (etiology, phenomenology, co-occurring disorders, treatment options, longitudinal course) for people with BPD was shown to result in significant improvements in a randomized controlled trial (Zanarini & Frankenburg, 2008), suggesting that this is likely to be an efficient strategy for time-strapped generalist clinicians.

9. Skills

In addition to content earlier in this chapter on DBT skills of mindfulness and emotion regulation, we have also included here information on two other DBT skills: distress tolerance skills and interpersonal effectiveness skills.

DBT distress tolerance skills

Linked with problem-solving, DBT clinicians often provide a simple psychoeducation paradigm to approaching a problem and related distress tolerance skills that many patients find helpful, as follows (Behavioral Tech licensed training):

- If can solve the problem, solve it.
- If can't solve the problem, try to feel better about the problem (distraction, self-soothing).
- If can't feel better about the problem, accept distress.

The goal that is explicitly shared with patients is that distress tolerance skills are less about permanently solving one's major life problems and more about getting through the situation without making things worse, say by overdosing or abusing one's landlord.

DBT interpersonal effectiveness skills

Many DBT patients value the structure and clarity of the acronym DEARMAN GIVE FAST, which is used to guide effective interpersonal assertiveness skills as follows:

Describe the situation

Express your feelings and opinions

Assert yourself

Reinforce the person ahead of time

be Mindful of objectives

Appear confident

Negotiate alternative solutions

Gentle

Interested

Validate the other person's feelings and opinions

Easy manner

Fair to ourselves

No overly **A**pologetic behavior

Stick to our values

Truthful

(Reproduced from Linehan, M. M. *The skills training manual for treating borderline personality disorder* © 1993, Guilford Press, with permission.)

Again, while this may seem obvious, it is often not the case for many of our patients, who often find the structure both novel and guiding.

All of the DEARMAN GIVE FAST skills can be used in any interpersonal situation with DEARMAN skills being to the fore where getting one's objective is the highest priority, GIVE skills to the fore when the quality of the relationship is highest priority, and FAST skills to the fore where self-respect is the highest priority.

10. Clinical feedback of treatment outcomes

A meta-analysis of mental health treatment outcome feedback studies reported a small but significant positive outcome ($p < 0.03$; $d = 0.10$) in favor of feedback in the short term (Knaup, Koesters, Schoefer, Becker, & Puschner, 2009). While a small effect on its own, in our opinion this size of change represents high value to overall outcome given the modest resources (time and cost) utilized. Randomized controlled trials have also demonstrated the value of such an approach reducing negative outcomes by over 50% and leading to improvements in client satisfaction and treatment alliance (Shimokawa, Lambert, & Smart, 2010). It is possible that a combination of improved therapeutic alliance and moderation of the wish to disengage from therapy accounts for some of the improvements observed. But what are the active ingredients of feedback? Moderator analyses showed that the effects were improved where feedback was recorded as progress (vs static), where both client and therapist received the feedback (vs one party only), and where the feedback was frequent (vs only once). This positive impact was not sustained in the few studies which had long-term follow-up after the end of the feedback intervention, suggesting either that feedback has no long-term effect or that feedback needs to be ongoing and continuous (Knaup et al., 2009). We believe the latter is the more plausible explanation, fitting with our clinical experience.

Feedback pathways that have utility in standard BPD generalist mental health practice include:

+ feedback from client verbally about symptoms, goals, treatment methods, and therapy relationship or via a simple individually created visual analogue scale

+ feedback from patients via a standardized scale such as the Outcome Rating Scale (Miller, Duncan, Brown, Sparks, & Claud, 2003) (readily available as below)

- freely available, very brief (1–2 minute) client-rated treatment outcome measures, including:

  - DASS 21 for depression, anxiety, and stress (Ng, Trauer, Dodd, Callaly, Campbell, & Berk, 2007; available from The University of New South Wales School of Psychology (www2.psy.unsw.edu.au))

  - DIM-10 for depression (Parker, Hilton, Bains, & Hadzi-Pavlovic, 2001; available from the Black Dog Institute website (www.blackdoginstitute. org.au, under "Depression in the medically ill"))

  - the Self-Compassion Scale short form for self-compassion (Raes, 2010; available from www.self-compassion.org).

MBT now uses a continuous feedback system on a sessional basis using a range of rapidly completed measures relevant to both patient and clinician. These include measures of quality of life, symptoms, social and interpersonal function, therapy process, and goal-based outcomes. The information is available to both patient and clinician for discussion in treatment. Feedback via tracking of targets daily by clients and weekly by therapists on a diary card is a standard part of DBT.

Research shows a sizable contribution of client expectancy of treatment outcome to psychotherapy treatment outcome (Norcross, 2002) replicated in people with BPD (Wenzel et al., 2008). Regular client feedback to the therapist (also collaboration, validation of negative client expectancy and behavioral and mentalizing experiments exploring alternative possibilities) is likely to be particularly helpful in improving the expectancy effect with patients who have a negative expectation of treatment outcome (Wenzel et al., 2008).

As treatment outcome feedback is beneficial, it seems highly plausible that alliance feedback will have a similar positive impact. The Session Rating Scale is an ultrabrief (15 second) visual analogue rating scale where the client rates the session at the end of it (Duncan et al., 2003; Duncan, 2003). The short version of the Working Alliance Inventory (Horvath & Greenberg, 1986) (WAI-SR) is used in MBT and is suitable for regular use with outpatients (Munder, Wilmers, Leonhart, Linster, & Barth, 2010).

Alliance feedback

The Session Rating Scale and the Outcome Rating Scale (see above) are both ultrabrief (15 seconds each) with obvious feasibility and utility advantages and satisfactory psychometrics given the ultrabrief nature of the scales. The two scales are readily and freely available for individuals and at a modest charge for organizations after registering with the Institute for the Study of Therapeutic Change at www.talkingcure.com. The Working Alliance Inventory is also readily available.

Epilogue

Consumer comment

Have hope—the statistics are on your side. I was once considered a hope-less case, but after skillful nonspecialist generalist mental health treatment am now working full time and leading an active social life. My journey of recovery has been like climbing a mountain. As I climbed higher, I discovered I was a strong, capable, and likeable woman. I have not reached all my goals yet but it is now several years since I self-harmed or even seriously considered it. I am now genuinely living a life with long-term goals and a vision for the future; something I didn't have before and didn't think was possible. All our journeys of recovery will be different, however my wish is that someone with BPD's journey will have been made a little easier for having read something in this book that will make a positive difference for you and thereby in turn for them (Jackson, personal communication).

Thank you for giving your energy and time to reading this book. We hope that the book has been of some benefit to you and will contribute in a small way to improving the quality of your clients' lives and the quality of your working life. The treatment of people with BPD is in an exciting era. In just over 20 years we have gone from a total absence of research evidence for effective treatments to broad evidence of a range of effective specialist treatments. Over the last few years this effectiveness research has started to extend to generalist treatments, the catalyst for this book. We hope that this book has translated some of the information from this research on generalist treatments into a useable format that has, or shortly will, resource you with practical, and clinically relevant, usable material that you can use to refine, and add to, your treatment of people with BPD. As a generalist mental health clinician you are important because most people with BPD are, and always will be, treated by generalist mental health clinicians like you. We would like to thank you for your interest in reading this book and for your enthusiasm for working with people with BPD. We have no doubt that people with BPD will be appreciative of your commitment and we hope that you also benefit from the work that you have done, and will continue to do, to improve the quality of lives of people with BPD. Best wishes in your future work in this era of increasing optimism about the treatment of BPD.

Anthony W. Bateman

Roy Krawitz

References

Abraham, P. F. & Calabrese, J. R. (2008). Evidence-based pharmacological treatment of borderline personality disorder: a shift from SSRIs to anticonvulsants and atypical antipsychotics? *Journal of Affective Disorders, 111,* 21–30.

Akiskal, H. S., Hirschfeld, R. M., & Yerevanian, B. I. (1983). The relationship of personality to affective disorders. *Archives of General Psychiatry, 40,* 801–810.

Allen, J. G., Fonagy, P., & Bateman, A. (2008). *Mentalizing in Clinical Practice* Washington, DC: APPI.

American Psychiatric Association (1994). *Diagnostic and Statistical Manual of Mental Disorders (DSM-IV)* (4th ed.). Washington, DC: American Psychiatric Association.

American Psychiatric Association (1998). Gold award: integrating dialectical behavior therapy into a community mental health program. *Psychiatric Services, 49,* 1138–1340.

American Psychiatric Association (2000). *Diagnostic and Statistical Manual of Mental Disorders. Text Revision (DSM-IV-TR)* (3rd (revised) ed.). Washington, DC: American Psychiatric Association.

American Psychiatric Association (2001). *Practice guideline for the treatment of patients with borderline personality disorder.* Washington DC: American Psychiatric Association. DOI: 10.1176/appi.books.

Appelbaum, A. H. (2006). Supportive psychoanalytic psychotherapy for borderline patients: an empirical approach. *American Journal of Psychoanalysis, 66,* 317–332.

Appelbaum, A. H. (2008). Supportive psychotherapy. *Journal of Lifelong Learning in Psychiatry, 3,* 438–449.

Arnsten, A. F. (1998). The biology of being frazzled. *Science, 280*(5370), 1711–1712.

Baron-Cohen, S. (2008) *Autism and Asperger Syndrome. The facts series.* Oxford: Oxford University Press.

Bartak, A., Andrea, H., Spreeuwenberg, M. D., Thunnissen, M., Ziegler, U. M., Dekker, J., et al. (2011). Patients with cluster a personality disorders in psychotherapy: an effectiveness study. [Comparative Study Controlled Clinical Trial Multicenter Study]. *Psychotherapy and Psychosomatics, 80*(2), 88–99.

Bartak, A., Andrea, H., Spreeuwenberg, M. D., Ziegler, U. M., Dekker, J., Rossum, B. V., et al. (2011). Effectiveness of outpatient, day hospital, and inpatient psychotherapeutic treatment for patients with cluster B personality disorders. [Clinical Trial Comparative Study Multicenter Study]. *Psychotherapy and Psychosomatics, 80*(1), 28–38.

Bartak, A., Spreeuwenberg, M. D., Andrea, H., Holleman, L., Rijnierse, P., Rossum, B. V., et al. (2010). Effectiveness of different modalities of psychotherapeutic treatment for patients with cluster C personality disorders: results of a large prospective multicentre study. [Multicenter Study]. *Psychotherapy and Psychosomatics, 79*(1), 20–30.

Bateman, A. (2011). Throwing the baby out with the bathwater. *Personality and Mental Health, 5,* 274–280.

Bateman, A. (2012). Treating borderline personality disorder in clinical practice. *American Journal of Psychiatry, 169,* 1–4.

Bateman, A. (2012). 100 words on mindfulness. *British Journal of Psychiatry, 201,* 297.

Bateman, A. & Fonagy, P. (1999). The effectiveness of partial hospitalization in the treatment of borderline personality disorder – a randomized controlled trial. *American Journal of Psychiatry, 156,* 1563–1569.

Bateman, A. & Fonagy, P. (2000). Effectiveness of psychotherapeutic treatment of personality disorder. *British Journal of Psychiatry, 177,* 138–143.

Bateman, A. & Fonagy, P. (2001). Treatment of borderline personality disorder with psychoanalytically oriented partial hospitalization: an 18-month follow-up. *American Journal of Psychiatry, 158,* 36–42.

Bateman, A. & Fonagy, P. (2003). Health service utilization costs for borderline personality disorder patients treated with psychoanalytically oriented partial hospitalization versus general psychiatric care. *American Journal of Psychiatry, 160,* 169–171.

Bateman, A. & Fonagy, P. (2004). *Psychotherapy for Borderline Personality Disorder: Mentalization-based treatment.* Oxford: Oxford University Press.

Bateman, A. & Fonagy, P. (2006). *Mentalization-based treatment: a practical guide.* Oxford: Oxford University Press.

Bateman, A. & Fonagy, P. (2008a). 8-year follow-up of patients treated for borderline personality disorder: mentalization-based treatment versus treatment as usual. *American Journal of Psychiatry, 165,* 631–638.

Bateman, A. & Fonagy, P. (2008b). Comorbid antisocial and borderline personality disorders: mentalization-based treatment. *Journal of Clinical Psychology: in session, 64,* 1–14.

Bateman, A. & Fonagy, P. (2009a). Psychotherapy for Personality Disorder. In M. G. Gelder, Lopez-Ibor, J. J. and Andreasen, N. C. (Ed.), *The New Oxford Textbook of Psychiatry* (2nd ed.) (pp. 892–900). Oxford: Oxford University Press.

Bateman, A. & Fonagy, P. (2009b). Randomized controlled trial of outpatient mentalization-based treatment versus structured clinical management for borderline personality disorder. *American Journal of Psychiatry, 1666,* 1355–1364.

Bateman, A. & Fonagy, P. (2012). *Handbook of mentalizing in mental health practice.* Washington, DC: American Psychiatric Press.

Beck, A. T. & Freeman, A. (1990). *Cognitive therapy of personality disorders.* New York: Guilford Press.

Betan, E., Heim, A., Conklin, C., & Westen, D. (2005). Countertransference phenomena and personality pathology in clinical practice: an empirical investigation. *American Journal of Psychiatry, 162,* 890–898.

Bevington, D. (2012). Supporting and enhancing mentalization in community outreach teams working with "hard to reach" youth: the AMBIT approach. In N. Midgley & I. Vrouva (Eds.), *Minding the Child: Mentalization-based interventions with children, young people and their families* (pp. 163–186). London: Routledge.

Black, D. W., Blum, N., Eichinger, L., McCormick, B., Allen, J., & Sieleni, B. (2008). STEPPS: Systems training for emotional predictability and problem solving in women offenders with borderline personality disorder in prison—a pilot study. *CNS Spectrum, 13,* 881–886.

Black, D. W., Gunter, T., Allen, J., Blum, N., Arndt, S., Wenman, G., et al. (2007). Borderline Personality Disorder in male and female offenders newly committed prison. *Comprehensive Psychiatry, 48,* 400–405.

Black, D. W., St John, D., Pfohl, B., McCormick, B., & Blum, N. (2009). Predictors of response to Systems Training for Emotional Predictability and Problem Solving (STEPPS) for borderline personality disorder: an exploratory study. *Acta Psychiatrica Scandinavica, 120,* 53–61.

Blum, N., St John, D., Pfohl, B., Stuart, S., McCormick, B., Allen, J., et al. (2008). Systems training for emotional predictability and problem solving (STEPPS) for outpatients with borderline personality disorder: a randomized controlled trial and 1-year follow-up. *American Journal of Psychiatry, 165,* 468–478.

Bohus, M., Landwehrmeyer, G., Stiglmayr, C., Limberger, M. F., Bohme, R., & Schmahl, C. (1999). Naltrexone in the treatment of dissociative symptoms in patients with borderline personality disorder: an open-label trial. *Journal of Clinical Psychiatry, 60,* 598–603.

Bornovalova, M. A., Hicks, B. M., Iacono, W. G., & McGue, M. (2009). Stability, change and heritability of borderline personality disorder traits from adolescence to adulthood: a longitudinal study. *Development and Psychopathology, 21,* 1335–1353.

Borschmann, R., Henderson, C., Hogg, J., Phillips, R., & Moran, P. (2012). Crisis interventions for people with borderline personality disorder (review). *Cochrane Database of Systematic Reviews.*

Bos, E. H., van Wel, E. B., Appelo, M. T., & Verbraak, M. J. (2010). A randomized controlled trial of a Dutch version of systems training for emotional predictability and problem solving for borderline personality disorder. *Journal of Nervous and Mental Disease, 198,* 299–304.

Bouchard, S., Sabourin, S., Lussier, Y., & Villeneuve, E. (2009). Relationship quality and stability in couples when one partner suffers from borderline personality disorder. *Journal of Marital and Family Therapy, 35,* 446–455.

Boutros, N., Torello, M., & McGlashan, T. (2003). Electrophysiological aberrations in borderline personality disorder: state of the evidence. *Journal of Neuropsychiatry and Clinical Sciences, 15,* 145–154.

Brassington, J. & Krawitz, R. (2006). Australasian dialectical behaviour therapy pilot outcome study: effectiveness, utility and feasibility. *Australasian Psychiatry, 14,* 313–319.

Brown, G. W., Birley, J. L. T., & Wing, J. K. (1972). Influence of family life on the course of schizophrenic disorders: a replication. *British Journal of Psychiatry, 121,* 241–258.

Brown, K. W., & Ryan, R. M. (2003). The benefits of being present: Mindfulness and its role in psychological well-being. *Journal of Personality and Social Psychology, 84,* 822–848.

Buteau, E., Dawkins, K., & Hoffman, P. (2008). In their own words: Improving services and hopefulness for families with BPD. *Social Work in Mental Health, 6,* 203–213.

Butzlaff, R. & Hooley, J. M. (1998). Expressed emotion and psychiatric relapse: a meta-analysis. *Archives of General Psychiatry, 55,* 547–552.

Carmody, J. & Baer, R. A. (2008). Relationships between mindfulness practice and levels of mindfulness, medical and psychological symptoms and well-being in a mindfulness-based stress reduction program. *Journal of Behavioral Medicine, 31,* 23–33.

Cecchin, G. (1987). Hypothesising, circularity and neutrality revisited: an invitation to curiosity. *Family Process,, 26*, 405–413.

Chan, A. O. M. & Silove, D. (2000). Nosological implications of psychotic symptoms in patients with established posttraumatic stress disorder. *Australian and New Zealand Journal of Psychiatry, 34*, 522–525.

Chanen, A. M., Jackson, H. J., McCutcheon, L. K., Jovev, M., Dudgeon, P., Yuen, H. P., et al. (2008). Early intervention for adolescents with borderline personality disorder using cognitive analytic therapy: randomised controlled trial. *British Journal of Psychiatry, 193*(6), 477–484.

Chanen, A. M., Jackson, H. J., McCutcheon, L. K., Jovev, M., Dudgeon, P., Yuen, H. P., et al. (2009). Early intervention for adolescents with borderline personality disorder: quasi-experimental comparison with treatment as usual. *Australian and New Zealand Journal of Psychiatry, 43*, 397–408.

Chanen, A. M., Jovev, M., & Jackson, H. J. (2007). Adaptive functioning and psychiatric symptoms in adolescents with borderline personality disorder. *Journal of Clinical Psychiatry, 68*, 297–306.

Chanen, A., McCutcheon, L., Germano, D., & Nistico, H. (2000). Good clinical care manual. Unpublished manuscript.

Chanen, A. M., McCutcheon, L. K., Germano, D., Nistico, H., Jackson, H. J., & McGorry, P. D. (2009). The HYPE Clinic: an early intervention service for borderline personality disorder. *Journal of Psychiatric Practice, 15*, 163–172.

Chiesa, M., Fonagy, P., Holmes, J., & Drahorad, C. (2004). Residential versus community treatment of personality disorders: a comparative study of three treatment program. *American Journal of Psychiatry, 161*, 1463–1470.

Chiesa, M., Fonagy, P., & Holmes, J. (2006). Six-year follow-up of three treatment programs to personality disorder. *Journal of Personality Disorders, 20*(5), 493–509.

Chiesa, M., Sharp, R., & Fonagy, P. (2011). Clinical associations of deliberate self-injury and its impact on the outcome of community-based and long-term inpatient treatment for personality disorder. *Psychotherapy and Psychosomatics, 80*, 100–109.

Clarke, D. (2003). Faith and hope. *Australasian Psychiatry 11:* 164–168.

Clarkin, J. F., Levy, K. N., Lenzenweger, M. F., & Kernberg, O. (2007). Evaluating three treatments for borderline personality disorder. *American Journal of Psychiatry, 164*, 922–928.

Coffey, S., Schumacher, J., Baschnagel, J., Hawk, L., Holloman, G., & Abraham, P. F. (2011). Impulsivity and risk-taking in borderline personality disorder with and without substance use disorders. *Personality Disorders: Theory, Research, and Treatment, 2*, 128–141.

Cohen, P., Chena, H., Crawford, T. N., Brook, J. S., & Gordon, K. (2007). Personality disorders in early adolescence and the development of later substance use disorders in the general population. *Drug and Alcohol Dependence, 88*, 71–84.

Colson, D. B., Allen, J., Coyne, L., Dexter, N., Jehl, N., Mayer, C. A., et al. (1986). An anatomy of countertransference: staff reactions to difficult psychiatric patients. *Hospital and Community Psychiatry, 37*, 923–928.

David, A., Hotopf, M., Moran, P., Owen, G., & Szmukler, G. (2010). Mentally disordered or lacking capacity? Lessons for management of serious deliberate self harm. *British Medical Journal, 341*, 587–589.

Distel, M. A., Trull, T. J., Derom, C. A., Thiery, E. W., Grimmer, M. A., Martin, N. G., et al. (2008). Heritability of borderline personality disorder features is similar across three countries. *Psychological Medicine, 38*, 1219–1229.

Dixon, I., Lucksted, A., Stewart, B., Burland, J., Brown, C. H., Postrado, L., et al. (2004). Outcomes of the peer-taught 12-week family-to-family education program for severe mental illness. *Acta Psychiatrica Scandinavica, 109*, 207–215.

Doering, S., Hörz, S., Rentrop, M., Fischer-Kern, M., Schuster, P., & Benecke, C. (2010). Transference-focused psychotherapy v. treatment by community psychotherapists for borderline personality disorder: randomised controlled trial. *British Journal of Psychiatry, 196*, 389–395.

Domes, G., Czieschnek, D., Weidler, F., Berger, C., Fast, K., & Herpertz, S. C. (2008). Recognition of facial affect in Borderline Personality Disorder. *Journal of Personality Disorder, 22*, 135–147.

Domes, G., Schulze, L., & Herpertz, S. C. (2009). Emotion recognition in borderline personality disorder – a review of the literature. *Journal of Personality Disorder, 23*, 6–19.

Dubo, E. D., Zanarini, M. C., Lewis, R. E., & Williams, A. A. (1997). Childhood antecedents of self-destructiveness in borderline personality disorder. *Canadian Journal of Psychiatry, 42*, 63–69.

Duncan, B. l., Miller, S. D., Sparks, J. A., Claud, D. A., Reynolds, L. R., Brown, J., et al. (2003). The Session Rating Scale: psychometric properties of a "working" alliance measure. *Journal of Brief Therapy, 3*, 3–11.

Dyck, M., Habel, U., Slodczyk, J., Schlummer, J., Backes, V., Schneider, F., et al. (2009). Negative bias in fast emotion discrimination in borderline personality disorder. *Psychological Medicine, 39*, 855–864.

Fertuck, E., Jekal, A., Song, I., Wyman, B., Morris, M., Wilson, S., et al. (2009). Enhanced "Reading the Mind in the Eyes" in borderline personality disorder compared to healthy controls. *Psychological Medicine, 39*, 1979–1988.

Flood, C., Byford, S., Hendersen, C., Leese, M., Thornicroft, G., Sutherby, K., et al. (2006). Joint crisis plans for people with psychosis: economic evaluation of a randomised controlled trial. *British Medical Journal, 333*, 729–729.

Fonagy, P. (2003). The development of psychopathology from infancy to adulthood. *Infant Mental Health Journal, 24*, 212–239.

Fonagy, P. & Bateman, A. (2006). Progress in the Treatment of Borderline Personality Disorder. *British Journal of Psychiatry, 188*, 1–3.

Fonagy, P. & Bateman, A. (2007). Mentalizing and borderline personality disorder. *Journal of Mental Health, 16*, 83–101.

Fonagy, P. & Bateman, A. (2008a). The development of borderline personality disorder—a mentalizing model. *Journal of Personality Disorders, 22*, 4–21.

Fonagy, P. & Bateman, A. (2008b). Attachment, mentalization and borderline personality disorder. *European Psychotherapy, 8*, 35–47.

Fonagy, P., Gergely, G., Elliot, J., & Target, M. (2002). Affect Regulation, Mentalization, and the Development of Self. London: Other Press.

Fonagy, P., Target, M., & Gergely, G. (2000). Attachment and borderline personality disorder: A theory and some evidence. *Psychiatric Clinics of North America, 23*, 103–122.

Frankenburg, F. R. & Zanarini, M. C. (2006). Obesity and obesity-related illnesses in borderline patients. *Journal of Personality Disorders, 20*(1), 71–80.

Franx, G., Kroon, H., & Grimshaw, J. (2008). Organizational change to transfer knowledge and improve qaulity and outcomes of care for patients with severe mental illness: a systematic overview of reviews. *Canadian Journal of Psychiatry (Revue Canadienne de Psychiatrie), 53*, 294–305.

Fruzzetti, A. E. & Iverson, K. M. (2006). Intervening with couples and families to treat emotion dysregulation and psychopathology. In D. K. Snyder, J. A. Simpson & J. N. Hughes (Eds.), *Emotion regulation in couples and families: pathways to dysfunction and health* (pp. 249–267). Washington, DC: American Psychological Association.

Fruzzetti, A. E., Santisteban, D. A., & Hoffman, P. H. (2007). Dialectical behavior therapy with families. In L. A. Dimeff & K. Koerner (Eds.), *Dialectical behavior therapy in clinical practice: applications across disorders and settings* (pp. 222–244). New York: Guilford Press.

Fruzzetti, A. E., Shenk, C., & Hoffman, P. D. (2005). Family interaction and the development of borderline personality disorder: a transactional model. *Development and Psychopathology, 17*, 1007–1030.

Gabbard, G., Coyne, L., Allen, J., Spohn, H., Colson, D., & Vary, M. (2000). Evaluation of intensive in-patient treatment of patients with severe personality disorders. *Psychiatric Services, 51*, 893–898.

Gergely, G. (2001). Kinds of Agents: The Origins of Understanding Instrumental and Communicative Agency. In U. Goshwami (Ed.), *Handbook of Childhood Cognitive Development* (pp. 54–62). Oxford: Blackwell.

Gieson-Bloo, J., van Dyck, R., Spinhoven, P., van Tilburg, W., Dirksen, C., van Asselt, T., et al. (2006). Outpatient psychotherapy for borderline personality disorder; randomized trial of schema-focused therapy vs transference-focused therapy. *Archives of General Psychiatry, 63*, 649–658.

Giffin, J. (2008). Family experience of borderline personality disorder. *Australian and New Zealand Journal of Family Therapy, 29*, 133–138.

Gilbert, P. (2009). *The compassionate mind.* London: Constable.

Gilbert, P. (2010). *Compassion focused therapy.* London: Routledge.

Goodman, M., Patil, U., Triebwasser, J., Diamond, E., Hiller, A., Hoffman, P., et al. (2010). Parental viewpoints of trajectories to borderline personality disorder in female offspring. *Journal of Personality Disorders, 24*, 204–216.

Grant, B. F., Chou, S. P., Goldstein, R. B., Huang, B., Stinson, F. S., Saha, T. D., et al. (2008). Prevalence, correlates, disability, and comorbidity of DSM-IV borderline personality disorder: results from the Wave 2 National Epidemiologic Survey on Alcohol and Related Conditions. *Journal of Clinical Psychiatry, 69*, 533–545.

Gratz, K. L. (2007). Targeting emotion dysregulation in the treatment of self-injury. *Journal of Clinical Psychology: In session, 63*, 1091–1103.

Greenberg, L. & Safran, J. (1987). *Emotion in Psychotherapy.* New York: Guilford Press.

Grepmair, L., Mitterlehner, F., Loew, T., Bachler, E., Rother, W., & Nickel, M. (2007). Promoting mindfulness in psychotherapists in training influences the treatment results of their patients: a randomized, double-blind, controlled study. *Psychotherapy and. Psychosomatics, 76*, 332–338.

Gunderson, J. & Phillips, K. (1991). A current view of the interface between borderline personality disorder and depression. *American Journal of Psychiatry, 148*, 967–975.

Gunderson, J. G. (2008). *Borderline Personality Disorder: A Clinical Guide (with Paul Links)*. Washington DC: American Psychiatric Publishing.

Gunderson, J. G. (2010). Revising the borderline diagnosis for DSM-V: an alternative proposal. [Research Support, N.I.H., Extramural]. *Journal of Personality Disorders, 24*(6), 694–708.

Gunderson, J. G., Berkowitz, C., & Ruiz-Sancho, A. (1997). Families of borderline patients: a psychoeducational approach. *Bulletin of the Menninger Clinic, 61*, 446–457.

Gunderson, J. G. & Lyons-Ruth, K. (2008). BPD's interpersonal hypersensitivity phenotype: a gene-environment-developmental model. *Journal of Personality Disorders, 22*, 22–41.

Gunderson, J. G., Morey, L. C., Stout, R. L., Skodol, A. E., Shea, M. T., McGlashan, T. H., et al. (2004). Major depressive disorder and borderline personality disorder revisited: longitudinal interactions. [Comparative Study Research Support, U.S. Gov't, P.H.S.]. *Journal of Clinical Psychiatry, 65*(8), 1049–1056.

Gunderson, J. G., Najavits, L.M., Leonhard, C., et al. (1997). Ontogeny of the therapeutic alliance in borderline patients. *Journal of Psychotherapy Reasearch, 7*, 301–309.

Gunderson, J. G., Stout, R. L., McGlashan, T. H., Shea, M. T., Morey, L. C., Grilo, C. M., et al. (2011). Ten-year course of borderline personality disorder: psychopathology and function from the collaborative longitudinal personality disorders study. *Archives of General Psychiatry*, 827–837.

Gunderson, J. G., Stout, R. L., Sanislow, C. A., Shea, M. T., McGlashan, T. H., Zanarini, M. C., et al. (2008). New episodes and new onsets of major depression in borderline and other personality disorders. [Research Support, N.I.H., Extramural]. *Journal of Affective Disorders, 111*(1), 40–45.

Gunderson, J. G., Weinberg, I., Daversa, M. T., Kueppenbender, K. D., Zanarini, M. C., Shea, M. T., et al. (2006). Descriptive and longitudinal observations on the relationship of borderline personality disorder and bipolar disorder. *American Journal of Psychiatry, 163*(7), 1173–1178.

Gurvitz, L., Koenigsberg, H., & Siever, L. (2000). Neurotransmitter dysfunction in patients with borderline personality disorder. *Psychiatric Clinics of North America, 23*, 27–40.

Gutheil, T. (1989). Borderline personality disorder, boundary violations, and patient-therapist sex: Medicolegal pitfalls. *American Journal of Psychiatry, 146*, 597–602.

Hahn, T. N. (1975). *The Miracle of Mindfulness: A Manual on Meditation*. Boston: Beacon Press.

Hamner, M. B., Frueh, C., Ulmer, H. G., & Arana, G. W. (1999). Psychotic features and illness severity in combat veterans with chronic posttraumatic stress disorder. *Biological Psychiatry, 45*, 846–852.

Hawton, K., Saunders, K., & O'Connor, R. (2012). Self-harm and suicide in adolescents. *Lancet, 379*, 2373–2382.

Henderson, C., Flood, C., Leese, M., Thornicroft, G., Sutherby, K., & Szmukler, G. (2004). Effect of joint crisis plans on use of compulsory treatment in psychiatry: single blind randomised controlled trial. *Social Psychiatry and Psychiatric Epidemiology, 44,* 369–337.

Henderson, C., Flood, C., Leese, M., Thornicroft, G., Sutherby, K., & Szmukler, G. (2009). Views of service users and providers on joint crisis plans: single blind randomized controlled trial. *British Medical Journal, 329,* 136–138.

Henry, C., Mitropoulou, V., New, A. S., Koenigsberg, H. W., Silverman, J., & Siever, L. J. (2001). Affective instability and impulsivity in borderline personality and bipolar II disorders: similarities and differences. *Journal of Psychiatric Research, 35,* 307–312.

Henry, W. P., Schacht, T. E., & Strupp, H. (1990). Patient and therapist introject, interpersonal process and differential outcome. *Journal of Consulting and Clinical Psychology, 58,* 768–774.

Herman, J. (1992). *Trauma and Recovery: from domestic abuse to political terror.* London: Harper Collins.

Herman, J. L., Perry, C., & van der Kolk, B. A. (1989). Childhood trauma in borderline personality disorder. *American Journal of Psychiatry, 146,* 490–495.

Hoffman, P. D., Fruzzetti, A. E., & Buteau, E. (2007). Understanding and engaging families: an education, skills and support program for relatives impacted by borderline personality disorder. *Journal of Mental Health, 16,* 69–82.

Hoffmann, P. D., Fruzzetti, A. E., Buteau, E., Neiditch, E. R., Penney, D., Bruce, M. L., et al. (2005). Family Connections: a program for relatives of persons with borderline personality disorder. *Family Process, 44,* 217–225.

Hoffman, P., Fruzzetti, A., & Swenson, C. (1999). Dialectical behavior therapy—family skills training. *Family Process, 38,* 399–414.

Hoffman, P. D. & Hooley, J. M. (1998). Expressed emotion and treatment of borderline personality disorder. In-session. *Psychotherapy in Practice, 4,* 39–54.

Hooley, J. M. & Hoffman, P. D. (1999). Expressed emotion and clinical outcome in borderline personality disorder. *American Journal of Psychiatry, 156,* 1557–1562.

Horvath, A. O. & Bedi, R. P. (2002). The alliance. In J. C. Norcross (Ed.), *Psychotherapy relationships that work* (pp. 37–69). Oxford: Oxford university Press.

Horvath, A. O. & Greenberg, L. (1986). The development of the Working Alliance Inventory: A research handbook. In L. Greenberg & W. Pinsoff (Eds.), *Psychotherapeutic Processes: A Research Handbook* (pp. 529–556). New York: Guilford Press.

Huband, N., McMurran, M., Evans, C., & Duggan, C. (2007). Social problem solving plus psychoeducation for adults with personality disorder: A pragmatic randomised controlled trial. *British Journal of Psychiatry, 190,* 307–313.

Huber, C. (2001). *There is nothing wrong with you: going beyond self-hate: a compassionate process for learning to accept yourself exactly as you are.* USA: Keep it Simple Books.

Ingenhoven, T., Lafay, P., Rinne, T., Passchier, J., & Duivenvoorden, H. (2010). Effectiveness of pharmacotherapy for severe personality disorders: meta-analyses of randomized controlled trials. *Journal of Clinical Psychiatry, 71,* 14–25.

Ivezic, S., Oruc, L., & Bell, P. (1999). Psychotic symptoms in post-traumatic stress disorder. *Military Medicine, 164,* 73–75.

Jacob, G. A., Guenzler, C., Zimmerman, S., Scheel, C. N., Rusch, N., Leonhart, R., et al. (2008). Time course of anger and other emotions in women with borderline personality disorder: a preliminary study. *Journal of Behavior Therapy, 39,* 391–402.

Jacob, G. A., Hellstern, K., Ower, N., Pillman, M., Scheel, C. N., Rusch, N., et al. (2009). Emotional reactions to standardized stimuli in women with borderline personality disorder: stronger negative affect, but no differences in reactivity. *Journal of Nervous and Mental Disease, 197,* 808–815.

James, W. (1890). *Principles of Psychology.* New York: Henry Holt & Co.

Joyce, P. R., McKenzie, J. M., Mulder, R. T., Luty, S. E., Sullivan, P. F., Miller, A. L., et al. (2006). Genetic, developmental and personality correlates of self-mutilation in depressed patients. *Australian and New Zealand Journal of Psychiatry, 40,* 225–229.

Jurist, E. J. (2005). Mentalized affectivity. *Psychoanalytic Psychology, 22,* 426–444.

Karterud, S. & Bateman, A. (2011). *Manual for mentaliseringsbasert psykoedukativ gruppeterapi.* Oslo: Gyldendal.

Keller, M. B., Lavori, P. W., Mueller, T. I., Endicott, J., Coryell, W., Hirschfeld, R. M., et al. (1992). Time to recovery, chronicity, and levels of psychopathology in major depression. A 5-year prospective follow-up of 431 subjects. *Archives of General Psychiatry, 49(10)(Oct),* 809–816.

King-Casas, B., Sharp, C., Lomax-Bream, L., Lohrenz, T., Fonagy, P., & Read Montague, P. (2008). The rupture and repair of cooperation in Borderline Personality Disorder. *Science, 321,* 806–810.

Knaup, C., Koesters, M., Schoefer, D., Becker, T., & Puschner, B. (2009). Effect of feedback of treatment outcome in specialist mental health care: meta-analysis. *British Journal of Psychiatry 195,* 15–22.

Koenigsberg, H. W., Harvey, P. D., Mitropoulou, V., Schmeidler, J., New, A. S., & Goodman, M. (2002). Characterizing affective instability in borderline personality disorder. *American Journal of Psychiatry, 159,* 784–788.

Kolla, N. J., Links, P. S., McMain, S., Streiner, D. L., Cardish, R., & Cook, M. (2009). Demonstrating adherence to guidelines for the treatment of patients with borderline personality disorder. *Canadian Journal of Psychiatry, 54,* 181–189.

Koons, C. R., Robins, C. J., Tweed, J. L., Lynch, T. R., Gonzalez, A. M., Morse, J. Q., et al. (2001). Efficacy of dialectical behavior therapy in women veterans with borderline personality disorder. *Behavior Therapy, 32,* 371–390.

Korzekwa, M. I., Dell, P. F., Links, P. S., Thabane, L., & Fougere, P. (2009). Dissociation in borderline personality disorder: a detailed look. *Journal of Trauma and Dissociation, 10,* 346–367.

Krawitz, R. (2004). Borderline personality disorder: attitudinal change following training. *Australian and New Zealand Journal of Psychiatry, 38,* 554–559.

Krawitz, R. (2008). *Borderline personality disorder: personal journeys of recovery, inspiration and hope.* Hamilton: Waikato District Health Board.

Krawitz, R. & Jackson, W. (2008). *Borderline personality disorder: the facts.* Oxford: Oxford University Press.

Krawitz, R. & Watson, C. (2003). *Borderline personality disorder: a practical guide to treatment.* Oxford: Oxford University Press.

Kuipers, L. (1979). Expressed emotion: a review. *British Journal of Social and Clinical Psychology(18),* 237–243.

Kuo, J. R. & Linehan, M. M. (2009). Disentangling emption processes in borderline personality disorder: physiological and self-reported assessment of biological vulnerability, baseline intensity, and reactivity to emotionally evocative stimuli. *Journal of Abnormal Psychology, 118,* 531–544.

Kvarstein, E. & Karterud, S. (2012). Large variations of global functioning over five years in treated patients with personality traits and disorders. *Journal of Personality Disorders, 26,* 141–161.

Lambert, M. J. & Barley, D. E. (2002). Research summary on the therapeutic relationship and psychotherapy. In J. C. Norcross (Ed.), *Psychotherapy relationships that work* (pp. 17–32). Oxford: Oxford University Press.

Laporte, L. & Guttman, H. (1996). Traumatic childhood experiences as risk factors for borderline and other personality disorders. *Journal of Personality Disorders, 10,* 247–259.

Lees, J., Manning, N., & Rawlings, B. (1999). *Therapeutic community effectiveness. A systematic international review of therapeutic community treatment for people with personality disorders and mentally disordered offenders.* NHS Centre for Reviews and Dissemination: University of York (CRD Report 17) http://www.york.ac.uk/inst/crd/CRD_Reports/crdreport17.pdf.

Leff, J., Kuipers, L., Berkowitz, R., Eberlein-Vries, R., & Sturgeon, D. (1982). A controlled trial of social intervention in the families of schizophrenia patients. *British Journal of Psychiatry, 141,* 121–134.

Leslie, A. M. (1987). Pretense and representation: The origins of "Theory of Mind." *Psychological Review, 94,* 412–426.

Levy, K. N., Meehan, K. B., Clarkin, J. F., Kernberg, O. F., Kelly, K. M., Reynoso, J. S., et al. (2006). Change in attachment patterns and reflective function in a randomized control trial of transference-focused psychotherapy for borderline personality disorder. *Journal of Consulting and Clinical Psychology, 74,* 1027–1040.

Lieb, K., Völlm, B., Rücker, G., Timmer, A., & Stoffers, J. (2010). Pharmacotherapy for borderline personality disorder: Cochrane systematic review of randomised trials. *British Journal of Psychiatry, 196,* 4–12.

Linehan, M. M. (1993a). *Cognitive-Behavioral Treatment of Borderline Personality Disorder.* New York: Guilford Press.

Linehan, M. (1993b). *The Skills Training Manual for Treating Borderline Personality Disorder.* New York: Guilford Press.

Linehan, M. M. (1997). *Validation and psychotherapy.* Washington, DC: American Psychological Association.

Linehan, M. M., Armstrong, H., Suarez, A., Allmon, D., & Heard, H. (1991). Cognitive-behavioral treatment of chronically parasuicidal borderline patients. *Archives of General Psychiatry, 48,* 1060–1064.

Linehan, M. M., Bohus, M., & Lynch, T. R. (2007). Dialectical behavior therapy for pervasive emotion dysregulation. In J. J. Gross (Ed.), *Handbook of emotion regulation* (pp. 581–605). New York: Guilford Press.

Linehan, M. M., Comtois, K. A., Murray, A. M., Brown, M. Z., Gallop, R. J., Heard, H. L., et al. (2006). Two-year randomized controlled trial and follow-up of dialectical behavior therapy vs therapy by experts for suicidal behaviors and borderline personality disorder. *Archives of General Psychiatry, 63*(7), 757–766.

Linehan, M. M., Dimeff, L., Reynolds, S. K., Comtois, K. A., Welch, S. S., Heagerty, P., et al. (2002). Dialectical behavior therapy versus comprehensive validation therapy plus 12-step for the treatment of opioid-dependent women meeting criteria for borderline personality disorder. *Drug and Alcohol Dependence, 67,* 13–26.

Linehan, M. M., Schmidt, H., Dimeff, L. A., Craft, J. C., Kanter, J., & Comtois, K. A. (1999). Dialectical behavior therapy for patients with borderline personality disorder and drug dependence. *American Journal on Addictions, 8,* 279–292.

Lingiardi, V., Filippucci, L., & Baiocco, R. (2005). Therapeutic alliance evaluation in personality disorders psychotherapy. *Psychotherapy Research, 15,* 45–54.

Lynch, T. R., Rosenthal, M. Z., Kosson, D. S., Cheavens, J. S., Lejuez, C. W., & Blair, R. J. (2006). Heightened sensitivity to facial expressions of emotion in borderline personality disorder. *Emotion, 6*(4), 647–655.

Magill, C. A. (2004). The boundary between borderline personality disorder and bipolar disorder: current concepts and challenges. *Canadian Journal of Psychiatry, 49,* 551–556.

Marsh, A. A. & Blair, R. J. (2008). Deficits in facial affect recognition among antisocial populations: a meta-analysis. *Neuroscience and Biobehavioral Reviews, 32,* 454–465.

Martin, D. J., Garske, J.P. and Katherine Davis, M. (2000). Relation of the therapeutic alliance with outcome and other variables: a meta-analytic review. *Journal of Consulting and Clinical Psychology, 68,* 438–450.

Mason, B. (1993). Towards positions of safe uncertainty. *Human Systems, 4,* 189–200.

McCloskey, M., New, A., Siever, L., Goodman, M., Koenigsberg, H., Flory, J., et al. (2011). Evaluation of behavioral impulsivity and aggression tasks as endophenotypes for borderline personality disorder. *Journal of Psychiatric Research, 43,* 1036–1048.

McFarlane, W. R., Dixon, L., Lukens, E., & Lucksted, A. (2003). Family psychoeducation and schizophrenia: a review of the literature. *Journal of Marital and Family Therapy, 29,* 223–245.

McMain, S., Guimond, T., Cardish, R., Streiner, D., & Links, P. (2012). Clinical outcomes and functioning post-treatment: a two-year follow-up of dialectical behavior therapy versus general psychiatric management for borderline personality disorder. *American Journal of Psychiatry, 169,* 650–661.

McMain, S., Links, P., Gnam, W., Guimond, T., Cardish, R., Korman, L., et al. (2009). A randomized controlled trial of dialectical behavior therapy versus general psychiatric management for borderline personality disorder. *American Journal of Psychiatry, 166,* 1365–1374.

Miller, J., Campbell, W., & Pilkonis, P. (2007). Narcissistic personality disorder: relations with distress and functional impairment. *Comprehensive Psychiatry, 48,* 170–177.

Miller, S. D., Duncan, B. L., Brown, J., Sparks, J., & Claud, D. (2003). The Outcome Rating Scale: A preliminary study of the reliability, validity, and feasibility of a brief visual analog measure. *Journal of Brief Therapy, 2,* 91–100.

Miller, W. R. & Rollnick, S. (2002). *Motivational interviewing.* New York: Guilford Press.

Moran, P., Borschmann, R., Flach, C., Barrett, B., Byford, S., Hogg, J., et al. (2010). The effectiveness of joint crisis plans for people with borderline personality disorder: protocol for an exploratory randomised controlled trial. *Trials* http://www.trialsjournal.com/content/11/1/18, *11.*

Munder, T., Wilmers, F., Leonhart, R., Linster, H. W., & Barth, J. (2010). Working Alliance Inventory-Short Revised (WAI-SR): psychometric properties in outpatients and inpatients. [Comparative Study]. *Clinical Psychology & Psychotherapy, 17*(3), 231–239.

Munroe-Blum, H. & Marziali, E. (1988). Time-limited group psychotherapy for borderline patients. *Canadian Journal of Psychiatry, 33,* 364–369.

Munroe-Blum, H. & Marziali, E. (1995). A controlled trial of short-term group treatment for borderline personality disorder. *Journal of Personality Disorders, 9,* 190–198.

Neacsiu, A. D., Rizvi, S. L., Vitaliano, P. P., Lynch, T. R., & Linehan, M. M. (2010). The dialectical behavior therapy ways of coping checklist: development and psychometric properties. *Journal of Clinical Psychology, 66*(6), 563–582.

Neff, K. D. & Vonk, R. (2009). Self-compassion versus global self-esteem: two different ways of relating to oneself. *Journal of Personality, 77,* 23–50w.

Newhill, C. E., Eack, S. M., & Mulvey, E. P. (2009). Violent behavior in borderline personality disorder. *Journal of Personality Disorders, 23,* 541–554.

Ng, F., Trauer, T., Dodd, S., Callaly, T., Campbell, S., & Berk, M. (2007). The validity of the 21-item version of the Depression Anxiety Stress Scales (DASS-21) as a routine clinical outcome measure. *Acta Neuropsychiatrica, 19,* 304–310.

NICE. (2009). Borderline Personality Disorder: treatment and management. http://www.nice.org.uk/Guidance/CG78/NiceGuidance/pdf/English.

Norcross, J. C. (2002). *Psychotherapy relationships that work.* Oxford: Oxford University Press.

Norris, D., Gutheil, T., & Strasburger, L. (2003). This couldn't happen to me: boundary problems and sexual misconduct in the psychotherapy relationship. *Psychiatric Services, 54,* 517–522.

Nose, M., Cipriani, A., Biancosino, B., Grassi, L., & Barbui, C. (2006). Efficacy of pharmacotherapy against core traits of borderline personality disorder: meta-analysis of randomized controlled trials. *International Journal of Clinical Psychopharmacology, 21,* 345–353.

Nunes, P. M., Wenzel, A., Borges, K. T., Porto, C. R., Caminha, R. M., & de Oliveira, I. R. (2009). Volumes of hippocampus and amygdala in patients with borderline personality disorder: a meta-analysis. *Journal of Personality Disorders, 23,* 333–345.

Ogata, S. N., Silk, K. R., & Goodrich, S. (1990). The childhood experience of the borderline patient. In P.Links (Ed.), *Family environment and borderline personality disorder* (pp. 87–103). Washington, DC: American Psychiatric Publishing.

Oldham, J. M., Bender, D. S., Skodol, A. E., Dyck, I. R., Sanislow, C. A., Yen, S., et al. (2004). Testing an APA practice guideline: symptom-targeted medication utilization for patients with borderline personality disorder. [Research Support, U.S. Gov't, P.H.S.]. *Journal of Psychiatric Practice, 10*(3), 156–161.

Oldham, J., Phillips, K., Gabbard, G., & Soloff, P. (2001). Practice Guideline for the Treatment of Patients with Borderline Personality Disorder. *American Journal of Psychiatry, 158,* 1–52.

Panksepp, J. (1998). *Affective neuroscience: The foundations of human and animal emotions.* New York: Oxford University Press.

Paris, J. (2003). Personality disorders over time: precursors, course and outcome. *Journal of Personality Disorders, 17,* 479–496.

Paris, J. (2004). Is hospitalization useful for suicidal patients with borderline personality disorder? *Journal of Personality Disorders, 18,* 240–247.

Paris, J. (2008). *Treatment of borderline personality disorder: a guide to evidence-based practice.* New York: Guilford Press.

Paris, J. (2010). Effectiveness of different psychotherapy approaches in the treatment of borderline personality disorder. *Current Psychiatry Reports, 12*, 56–60.

Paris, J. & Zweig-Frank, H. (2001). A 27-year follow-up of patients with borderline personality disorder. *Comprehensive Psychiatry, 42*, 482–487.

Parker, G., Hilton, T., Bains, J., & Hadzi-Pavlovic, D. (2001). Cognitive –based measures screening for depression in the medically ill: The DMI-10 and DMI-18. *Acta Psychiatrica Scandinavica, 105*, 419–426.

Pirkis, J., Burgess, P., Hardy, J., Harris, M., Slade, T., & Johnston, A. (2012). Who cares? A profile of people who care for relatives with a mental disorder. *Australian and New Zealand Journal of Psychiatry, 44*, 929–937.

Pitman, A., Krysinska, K., Osborn, D., & King, M. (2012). Suicide in young men. *Lancet, 379*, 2383–2392.

Porr, V. (2010). *Overcoming borderline personality disorder: a family guide for healing and change.* Oxford: Oxford University Press.

Powers, M. B., Zm Vorde Sive Vording, M., & Emmelkamp, P. M. G. (2009). Acceptance and commitment therapy: a meta-analytic review. *Psychotherapy and Psychosomatics, 78*, 73–80.

Prochaska, J. O., Norcross, J. C., & Diclemente, C. C. (1994). *Changing for good.* New York: Harper Collins.

Raes, F. (2010). Rumination and worry as mediators of the relationship between self-compassion and depression and anxiety. *Personality and Individual Differences, 48*, 757–761.

Rajalin, M., Wickholm-Pethrus, L., Hursti, T., & Jokinen, J. (2009). Dialectical behavior therapy-based skills training for family members of suicide attempters. *Archives of Suicide Research, 13*, 257–263.

Rathus, J. H. & Miller, A. L. (2002). DBT adapted for suicidal adolescents. *Suicide and Life-threatening Behavior, 32*, 146–157.

Rockland, L. H. (1992). *Supportive therapy for borderline patients: a psychodynamic approach.* New York: Guilford Press.

Roemer, E. & Orsillo, S. M. (2008). *Mindfulness-and acceptance-based behavioral therapies in practice: guides to individualized evidence-based treatments.* New York: Guilford Press.

Rogers, C. R. (1986). *Client-centered therapy.* San Francisco: Jossey-Bass.

Rosenthal, M. Z., Gratz, K. L., Cheavens, J. S., Lejuez, C. W., & Lynch, T. R (2008). Borderline personality disorder and emotional responding: a review of the research literature. *Clinical Psychology Review, 28*, 75–91.

Safran, J. D. & Muran, J. C. (2000). *Negotiating the therapeutic alliance: A relational treatment guide.* New York: Guilford Press.

Sanislow, C. A., Grilo, C. M., Morey, L. C., Bender, D. S., Skodol, A. E., & Gunderson, J. (2002). Confirmatory factor analysis of DSM-IV criteria for borderline personality disorder: findings from the collaborative longitudinal personality disorders study. *American Journal of Psychiatry, 159*, 284–290.

Sansone, R. A., Rytwinski, D., & Gaither, G. A. (2003). Borderline personality and psychotropic medication prescription in an outpatient psychiatry clinic. *Comprehensive Psychiatry, 44*, 454–458.

Saunders, E. F. & Silk, K. (2009). Personality trait dimensions and the pharmacological treatment of borderline personality disorder. *Journal of Clinical Psychopharmacology, 29*, 461–467.

Sautter, F. J., Brailey, K., Uddo, M. M., Hamilton, M. F., Beard, M. G., & Borges, A. H. (1999). PTSD and comorbid psychotic disorder: comparison with veterans diagnosed with PTSD or psychotic disorder. *Journal of Traumatic Stress, 12*, 73–88.

Schwartz, M. A. (1991). The nature and classification of the personality disorders: A reexamination of basic premises. *Journal of Personality Disorders, 5*, 25–30.

Shearin, E. N. & Linehan, M. M. (1994). Dialectical behavior therapy for borderline personality disorder: theoretical and empirical foundations. *Acta Psychiatrica Scandinavica, 89*, 61–68.

Shimokawa, K., Lambert, M. J., & Smart, D. W. (2010). Enhancing treatment outcome of patients at risk of treatment failure: meta-analytic and mega-analytic review of a psychotherapy quality assurance system. *Journal of Consulting and Clinical Psychology, 78*, 298–311.

Silk, K. (2008). Augmenting psychotherapy for borderline personality disorder: the STEPPS program. *American Journal of Psychiatry, 165*, 413–415.

Silk, K. R. & Jibson, M. D. (2010). Personality disorders. In A. J. Rothschild (Ed.), *The Evidence-Based Guide to Antipsychotic Medications* (pp. 101–124). Washington, DC: American Psychiatric Publishing.

Skodol, A. E., Bender, D. S., Morey, L. C., Clark, L. A., Oldham, J. M., Alarcon, R. D., et al. (2011). Personality disorder types proposed for DSM-5. *Journal of Personality Disorders, 25*(2), 136–169.

Skodol, A. E., Gunderson, J. G., Pfohl, B., Widiger, T. A., Livesley, W. J., & Siever, L. J. (2002). The borderline diagnosis I: psychopathology, comorbidity, and personality structure. *Biological Psychiatry, 51*(12), 936–950.

Skodol, A. E., Stout, R. L., McGlashan, T. H., Grilo, C. M., Gunderson, J., & Shea, M. T. (1999). Co-occurance of mood and personality disorders: a report from the Collaborative Longitudinal Personality Disorders Study (CLPS). *Depression and Anxiety, 10*, 175–182.

Soloff, P., Cornelius, J., & George, A. (1993). Efficacy of phenelzine and haloperidol in borderline personality disorder. *Archives of General Psychiatry, 50*, 377–385.

Steering-Committee. (2002). Empirically supported therapy relationships: conclusions and recommendations of the Division 29 Task Force. In J. C. Norcross (Ed.), *Psychotherapy relationships that work* (pp. 441–443). Oxford: Oxford University Press.

Stoffers, J., Vollm, B. A., Rucker, G., Timmer, A., Huband, N., & Lieb, K. (2010). Pharmacological interventions for borderline personality disorder. *Cochrane Database of Systematic Reviews, 6*, CD005653.

Stone, M. H. (1989). Long-term follow-up of narcissistic borderline patients. *Psychiatric Clinics of North America, 12*, 621–641.

Stone, M. H. (1990). *The fate of borderline patients: Successful outcome and psychiatric practice.* New York: Guilford Press.

Stone, M. H. (2006). Relationship of borderline personality disorder and bipolar disorder. *American Journal of Psychiatry, 163*, 1126–1128.

Swartz, M., Balzer, D., George, L., & Winfield, I. (1990). Estimating the prevalence of borderline personality disorder in the community. *Journal of Personality Disorders, 4*, 257–272.

Torgersen, S., Lygren, S., Oien, P., Skre, I., Onstad, S., Edvardsen, J., et al. (2000). A twin study of personality disorders. *Comprehensive Psychiatry, 41*, 416–425.

Trull, T. J., Sher, K. J., Minks-Brown, C., Durbin, J., & Burr, R. (2000). Borderline personality disorder and substance use disorders: a review and integration. *Clinical Psychology Review, 20*, 235–253.

Tryon, G. S. & Winograd, G. (2002). Goal consensus and collaboration. In J. C. Norcross (Ed.), *Psychotherapy relationships that work* (pp. 109–125). Oxford: Oxford University Press.

Turner, R. M. (2000). Naturalistic evaluation of dialectical behavior therapy-oriented treatment for borderline personality disorder. *Cognitive and Behavioral Practice, 7*, 413–419.

Tyrer, P. & Bateman, A. (2004). Drug treatment for personality disorder. *Advances in Psychiatric Treatment, 10*, 389–398.

Tyrer, P., Crawford, M., Mulder, R., Blashfield, R., Farnam, A., Fossati, A., et al. (2011). The rationale for the reclassification of personality disorder in the 11th revision of the International Calssification of Diseases (ICD-11). *Personality and Mental Health, 5*, 246–259.

Umgvari, G. S. & Mullen, P. E. (2000). Reactive psychoses revisited. *Australian and New Zealand Journal of Psychiatry, 34*, 458–467.

Van den Bosch, L. M. C., Koeter, M. W. J., Stijnen, T., Verhuel, R., & van den Brink, W. (2005). Sustained efficacy of dialectical behaviour therapy for borderline personality disorder. *Behavior Research and Therapy, 43*, 1231–1241.

Van den Bosch, L. M. C., Verhuel, R., Schippers, G. M., & van den Brink, W. (2002). Dialectical behavior therapy of borderline patients with and without substance use problems: implementation and long-term effects. *Addictive Behaviors, 27*, 911–923.

van Wel, B., Kockmann, I., Blum, N., Pfohl, B., Black, D. W., & Heesterman, W. (2006). STEPPS group treatment for borderline personality disorder in The Netherlands. *Annals of Clinical Psychiatry, 18*, 63–67.

Vaughn, C., N. & Leff, J. P. (1976). The influence of family and social factors on the course of psychiatric illness. *British Journal of Psychiatry, 129*, 125–137.

Verheul, R., Van Den Bosch, L. M., Koeter, M. W., De Ridder, M. A., Stijnen, T., & Van Den Brink, W. (2003). Dialectical behaviour therapy for women with borderline personality disorder: 12-month, randomised clinical trial in The Netherlands. *British Journal of Psychiatry, 182*, 135–140.

Vermote, R., Fonagy, P., Vertommen, H., Verhaest, Y., Stroobants, R., & Vandeneede, B. (2009). Outcome and outcome trajectories of personality disordered patients during and after a psychoanalytic hospitalization-based treatment. *Journal of Personality Disorder, 23*, 293–306.

Weinberg, I., Ronningstam, E., Goldblatt, M. J., Schechter, M., & Maltsberger, J. T. (2011). Common factors in empirically supported treatments of borderline personality disorder. *Current Psychiatry Reports, 13*, 60–68.

Wenzel, A., Jeglic, E. L., Levy-Mack, H. J., Beck, A. T., & Brown, G. K. (2008). Treatment attitude and therapy outcome in patients with borderline personality disorder. *Journal of Cognitive Psychotherapy, 22*, 250–257.

Whisman, M. A. & Schonbrun, Y. C. (2009). Social consequences of borderline personality disorder symptoms in a population-based survey: marital distress, marital violence and marital disruption. *Journal of Personality Disorders, 23*, 410–415.

Widiger, T. A. & Frances, A. J. (1989). Epidemiology, diagnosis and comorbidity of borderline personality disorder. In A. Tasman, R. E. Hales, & A. J. Frances (Eds.), *Review of Psychiatry* (pp. 8–24). Washington, DC: American Psychiatric Publishing.

Widiger, T. A. & Weissman, M. M. (1991). Epidemiology of borderline personality disorder. *Hospital and Community Psychiatry, 42*, 1015–1020.

Widom, C. S., Czaja, S. J., & Paris, J. (2009). A prospective investigation of borderline personality disorder in abused and neglected children followed up into adulthood. *Journal of Personality Disorders, 23*, 433–446.

Wright, J. H., Basco, M. R., & Thase, M. E. (2006). *Learning cognitive-behavior therapy: an illustrated guide*. Washington, DC: American Psychiatric Publishing.

Wupperman, P., Neumann, C. S., & Axelrod, S. R. (2008). Do deficits in mindfulness underlie borderline personality features and core difficulties? *Journal of Personality Disorders, 22*, 466–482.

Wupperman, P., Neumann, C. S., Whitman, J. B., & Axelrod, S. R. (2009). The role of mindfulness in borderline personality disorder features. *Journal of Nervous and Mental Disease, 10*, 766–771.

Yee, L., Korner, J., McSwiggan, S., Meares, R. A., & Stevenson, J. (2005). Persistent hallucinosis in borderline personality disorder. *Comprehensive Psychiatry, 46*, 147–154.

Zanarini, M. C. (2004). Update on pharmacotherapy of borderline personality disorder. [Research Support, U.S. Gov't, P.H.S. Review]. *Current Psychiatry Reports, 6*(1), 66–70.

Zanarini, M. C. (2008). Reasons for change in borderline personality disorder (and other axis II disorders). [Research Support, N.I.H., Extramural Review]. *The Psychiatric Clinics of North America, 31*(3), 505–515, viii.

Zanarini, M. C. (2009). Psychotherapy of borderline personality disorder. *Acta Psychiatrica Scandinavica, 120*, 373–377.

Zanarini, M. C., Frankenburg, F. R., Weingeroff, J. L., Reich, D. B., Fitzmaurice, G. M., & Weiss, R. D. (2011). The course of substance use disorders in patients with borderline personality disorder and Axis II comparison subjects: a 10-year follow-up study. [Research Support, N.I.H., Extramural]. *Addiction, 106*(2), 342–348.

Zanarini, M. C. & Frankenburg, F. R. (2003). Omega-3 fatty acid treatment of women with borderline personality disorder. *American Journal of Psychiatry, 160*, 167–169.

Zanarini, M. C. & Frankenburg, F. R. (2008). A preliminary, randomized trial of psychoeducation for women with borderline personality disorder. [Randomized Controlled Trial Research Support, Non-U.S. Gov't]. *Journal of Personality Disorders, 22*(3), 284–290.

Zanarini, M. C., Frankenburg, F. R., Dubo, E., Sickel, A., Trikha, A., Levin, A., et al. (1998). Axis I comorbidity of borderline personality disorder. *American Journal of Psychiatry, 155*, 1733–1739.

Zanarini, M. C., Frankenburg, F. R., Hennen, J., Bradford Reich, D., & Silk, K. (2004). Axis I comorbidity in patients with borderline personality disorder: 6-year follow-up and prediction of time to remission. *American Journal of Psychiatry, 161*, 2108–2114.

Zanarini, M. C., Frankenburg, F. R., Hennen, J., Reich, D. B., & Silk, K. R. (2004). Axis I comorbidity in patients with borderline personality disorder: 6-year follow-up and prediction of time to remission. [Comparative Study Research Support, U.S. Gov't, P.H.S.]. *American Journal of Psychiatry, 161*(11), 2108–2114.

Zanarini, M. C., Frankenburg, F. R., Hennen, J., & Silk, K. (2003). The longitudinal course of borderline psychopathology: 6-year prospective follow-up of the phenomenology of borderline personality disorder. *American Journal of Psychiatry, 160*, 274–283.

Zanarini, M. C., Frankenburg, F. R., Reich, D. B., & Fitzmaurice, G. (2010a). The 10-year course of psychosocial functioning among patients with borderline personality disorder and Axis II comparison subjects. [Comparative Study Research Support, N.I.H., Extramural]. *Acta Psychiatrica Scandinavica, 122*(2), 103–109.

Zanarini, M. C., Frankenburg, F. R., Reich, D. B., & Fitzmaurice, G. (2010b). Time to attainment of recovery from borderline personality disorder and stability of recovery: A 10-year prospective follow-up study. [Research Support, N.I.H., Extramural]. *American Journal of Psychiatry, 167*(6), 663–667.

Zanarini, M. C., Frankenburg, F. R., Reich, D., & Fitzmaurice, G. (2012). Attainment and stability of sustained symptomatic remission and recovery among patients with borderline personality disorder and Axis II comparison subjects: A 16-year prospective follow-up study. *American Journal of Psychiatry, 169*, 476–483.

Zanarini, M. C., Frankenburg, F. R., Reich, D. B., Fitzmaurice, G., Weinberg, I., & Gunderson, J. G. (2008). The 10-year course of physically self-destructive acts reported by borderline patients and axis II comparison subjects. [Comparative Study Research Support, N.I.H., Extramural]. *Acta Psychiatrica Scandinavica, 117*(3), 177–184.

Zanarini, M. C., Frankenburg, F. R., Reich, D. B., Marino, M. F., Haynes, M. C., & Gunderson, J. G. (1999). Violence in the lives of adult borderline patients. *Journal of Nervous and Mental Disease, 187*, 65–71.

Zanarini, M. C., Ruser, T., Frankenberg, F. R., & Hennen, J. (2000). The dissociative experiences of borderline patients. *Comprehensive Psychiatry, 41*, 223–227.

Zanarini, M. C., Williams, A. A., Lewis, R. E., Reich, R. B., Vera, R. C., Marino, M. F., et al. (1997). Reported pathological childhood experiences associated with the development of borderline personality disorder. *American Journal of Psychiatry, 154*, 1101–1106.

Zimmerman, M. & Mattia, J. I. (1999). Axis I diagnostic comorbidity and borderline personality disorder. *Comprehensive Psychiatry, 40*, 245–252.

Index

Note: page numbers in *italics* refer to figures

abandonment 8–9
absolutist thinking 16–17, 191–2
abuse 154
  involvement of family members/friends
    149
  see also child abuse; sexual abuse
acceptance 184–7
acceptance and commitment therapy 179
accountability 161
active clinicians 49–50, 83
active passivity 18–19
acute suicide risk 124, 129–30
  see also suicidal behavior; suicide risk;
    suicides
addictions *see* substance abuse
adherence monitoring 50–1
adolescents
  BPD diagnosis 4–5
  DBT parenting skills intervention 171
  duration of treatment 50
  family involvement 145
  I-BAFT 171
  MBT-A 171
advocacy 89–90
affective disorders
  co-occurrence with BPD 131
  see also bipolar affective disorder;
    depression
affective instability 11
agent-attribute propositions 87
agoraphobia 19, 98
alcohol abuse 20, 76, 132
Allen, J.G. et al. 53
alliance feedback 202
alliance ruptures 48
  management 75
  risks 129, 133
all-or-nothing thinking 16–17, 191–2
amnesic periods 13, 22
amygdala 23, 153
anger 182
  DSM-IV-TR diagnostic criterion 12
antipsychotic medication 136
  duration of use 141
  see also prescribing
antisocial personality disorder
  co-occurrence with BPD 23

perceptions of facial expression 104
anxiety management 97–8
Appelbaum, A. 41, 47, 48
Arnsten, A.F. 181
assessment 59–63, 77
see also medication review; risk assessment
attachment relationships 99
  discussion with family members 154
attachment system hyper-responsiveness 15
attempted suicide *see* self-harm
attention deficit hyperactivity disorder 20
attitude of the clinician 82–6
attributing personally 190
auditory hallucinosis 22
authenticity of the clinician 83–4
automatic thoughts 97
avoidant personality disorder 22–3
awareness of BPD 58

Baron-Cohen, S. 86–7
Bartak, A. et al. 126
Bateman, A. and Fonagy, P. 41–2, 48, 51,
    54–5, 115–16, 133, 176, 198
Bateman, A. et al. 39, 39–40, 47
Beck, A.T. 16
behavioral analysis *see* chain analysis
Bergmans, Y. 40
binge-eating disorder 20
biological vulnerability theory 14
bipolar affective disorder 19, 21, 99, 131
Black, D.W. et al. 169
black-and-white thinking 16–17, 191–2
Blum N. et al. 169
Bockian, N.R. et al. 165
Bolton, R. 39
borderline personality disorder (BPD)
  alternative names 6
  BPD traits 4
  co-occurring conditions 19–23
  diagnosis 4–5
    communication to the patient 63–4
    DSM-IV-TR diagnostic criteria 6–13
    screening questions 7–8
  epidemiology 3–4
  etiology 23–6, 152–5
  historical background 2–3
  identity issues 60

borderline personality (*Continued*)
  impulsivity 60–1
  interpersonal sensitivity 62
  prognosis 29–31, 155
  relationship difficulties 61–2
  suicidal behavior 20–1
  understanding of 13–19
"borderline voices" 22
Bornovalova, M.A. 153
Bos, E.H. et al. 169
boundary problems 113–14
brain, altered anatomy and function 23
Brown, K.W. & Ryan, R.M. 176
bulimia 20
Buteau, E. et al. 146, 155

cannabis use 132
  see also substance abuse
capacity/incapacity legislation 69–70
care program meetings 58
Carmody, J. & Baer, R.A. 53
Carsky, M. 41
case managers 138
case presentation 121
catastrophizing 190–1
causes of BPD 23–6, 152–5
Cecchin, G. 160
chain analysis 54, 193–7
  consumer comments 197–8
  of emotions 100
  of self-harm 111
challenges to the clinician 84
Chanen, A.M. et al. 5, 36, 40, 41
changeability, belief in 161
Chiesa, M. et al. 126
child abuse 4, 24–5, 26, 154
  involvement of family members/friends 149
Clarke, D. 190
Clarkin, J.F. et al. 41
clinical planning, teamwork 117–18
clinician errors 85–6
clinician monitoring 50–1
clinicians
  active 49–50
  attitude 44–5, 82–5
  fostering of therapeutic alliance 75
  responsibilities 72–3
  self-observation 52–3
  supervision of 51–2
  team support 113–14
  worry about patients 133–4
Coffey, S. et al. 61
cognitive analytic therapy 33, 41
cognitive behavioral therapy (CBT) 32
cognitive distortions 71
cognitive modification 188–92
Cohen, P. et al. 76
coherence of treatment models 51

Colson, D.B. et al. 133–4
commitment, acceptance and commitment
    therapy 179
commonalities across generalist treatments
    36–9, *37–8*
  aspects of treatment
    initial therapeutic stance 44–6
    therapy relationship 46–9
    treatment model features 49–53
  client self-observation 53–4
  language use 43
  method of determination 43
communication 58
comorbidities 19–21, 98–9, 130–2
  prescribing for 141
  substance abuse 76
compassionate attitude, clinicians 45, 47–8
competence, fluctuating 18
complex post-traumatic stress disorder 6
coordination of treatment 58, 114–15
core schemas 16
core treatment strategies
  advocacy 89–90
  clinician attitude 82–6
  empathy 86–7
  interviewing 81–2
  positive regard 88–9
  problem-solving groups 90–8
  validation 87–8
countertransference 52–3
countervalent expression strategies 96
couples
  DBT skills intervention 171
  see also partners
crisis planning 65
  consumer comments 68, 198–9
  joint crisis plans 198
  management 138–9
    what can other people do and not do? 66
    what can services do and not do? 67
    what can the patient do and not do? 66
  for self-harm 111
  for suicidal behavior 129
  telephone contact 73
  warning signs, identification of 65–6
criticism 117
curiosity 160
cutting *see* self-harm

DASS 21 201
David, A. et al. 69
DBT *see* dialectical behavior therapy (DBT)
DEARMAN GIVE FAST skills 200–1
"de-fusion" 187, 188
demoralization, team support 118–19
dependent personality disorder 22–3
depersonalization 22
depression 19, 21, 98–9, 131

selective serotonin reuptake inhibitors 136
derealization 22
devaluation 9
diagnosis 4–5, 58
 advantages and disadvantages 5
 communication to the patient 63–4
 consumer comment 5
 discriminating features 13
 DSM-IV-TR diagnostic criteria 6–14
 DSM-V classification 2–3, 6
 female predominance 3–4, 26
 screening questions 7–8
dialectical behavior therapy (DBT) 24, 153–4
 accepting thoughts and valued action
  187–8
 chain analysis 194
 comparison with general psychiatric
  management 40
 comparison with SP and transference-
  focused psychotherapy 41
 DBT Family Skills Training 170
 decreasing hyperarousal 192–3
 distress tolerance skills 200
 feedback 202
 interpersonal effectiveness skills 200–1
 reading list 164–5
 skills acquisition 55
 teamwork 113
 treatment outcome studies 32
 "turning the mind" 185
 validation 159
dichotomous thinking 16–17, 191–2
DIM-10 202
discussion, team meetings 121
dissociative symptoms 12–13, 20, 22
Distel, M.A. et al. 24, 153
distraction techniques 97–8
distress
 reduction by self-harm 27–9
 valued action 184
distress tolerance skills 200
divalproex sodium 136
Division 29 Task Force on Empirically
 Supported Therapy Relationships
 46–7
Dixon, I. et al. 147
Dobbs, B. 164
drop-out, relationship to therapeutic
 alliance 74
drug abuse *see* substance abuse
Duncan, B.I. et al. 202
duration of treatment 50
Dyck, M. et al. 50
dysthymic disorder 19, 21, 99

earnings gaps, relationship to BPD prevalence 3
eating disorders 20
emergency appointments 67

emergency services, role in crisis
 management 67
emotional dysregulation 6, 61, 71
emotional instability 11
emotional intensity disorder 6
emotional sensitivity 14–15, 24
 explanation to family members 153–4
 group discussions 104–5
emotion group, DSM-IV-TR diagnostic
 criteria 14
emotions
 acceptance of 181–3
 avoidance of 9
 chain analysis 100
 decreasing hyperarousal 192–3
 functions 181–2
 group discussions 92–8
 identification of 54, 95, 100–1, 182–3
 link to interpersonal interactions 99–100
 primary and secondary 94–5, 184
 "Riding the Wave" 183
 as signals 100
empathy 23, 47–8, 49, 86–7
 family/friend interventions 155–7
emptiness, feelings of 11–12
enthusiasm, clinicians 44–5
errors, clinicians' 85–6
escalator scale, crises 66
etiology of BPD 23–6, 152–5
events analysis 54
experts in BPD, effective treatment
 recommendations 41–3
"expressed emotion" 148

facial expressions, patient perceptions 83, 104
fallibility 192
family connections, protection against BDP 3
Family Connections program 150–1, 169–70
family/friend interventions 78–9, 144–5
 BPD handout 172–3
 consumer comment 161
 etiological understanding 152–5
 guidance 149
 hope, provision of 155
 multisession interventions 166–8
 NICE guidelines 145
 outcome research 169–71
 rationale 145–7
 reading list 164–5
 relationship to outcome 148
 self-care 162–3
 short intervention 150–1
 summary 142–3
 teaching mentalization skills 160–1
 teaching positive reinforcement 162
 teaching validation and empathy skills
  155–9
 useful websites 165–6

family/friends, impact of BPD 146–7
"Family-to-family" program 147
fear 182
feasibility studies, psychosocial treatment 33
feedback 201–2
feelings
  group discussions 92–8
  see also emotions
female predominance of BPD diagnosis 3–4, 26
Fertuck, E. et al. 83
"flashback" experiences 22
Flood, C. et al. 198
fluvoxamine 136
focus for treatment 51, 58
follow-up 152
Fonagy, P. 15, 39
Fonagy, P. & Bateman, A. 128
forgiveness 160
formulation 77–8
Friedel, R.O. 165
  website 166
friends *see* family/friend interventions
Fruzzetti, A.E. 156, 164, 168, 171
Fruzzetti, A.E. & Iverson, K.M. 170
functional analysis *see* chain analysis

Gabbard, G. 83, 127
generalist treatments 34–6
  commonalities 36–9, *37–8*
    aspects of treatments 44–53
    client self-observation 53–4
    language use 43
    method of determination 43
  general psychiatric management 40
  good clinical care 40–1
  structured clinical management 39–40
  supportive psychotherapy 41
  treatment details, sources 43
generalized anxiety disorder 19
general psychiatric management (GPM) 40
genetic factors in BPD 24–5, 153
Germano, D. 40
Giffin, J. 146
Gilbert, P. 192, 193
good clinical care (GCC) 40–1
  family/friend interventions 144
Goodman, M. et al. 153
Grant, B.F. et al. 26
Grepmair, L. et al. 53
grief, "positive grieving" 151–2
group discussions
  problem-solving approach 90
    impulse control 101–3
    mood regulation 98–101
    practical problems 90
    self-harm 105–11
    sensitivity and interpersonal problems
      104–5

symptoms reduction 92
  tolerance of emotions 92–8
  of self-harm 105–11
  teamwork 120
guilt, feelings of, family members 152, 153
Gunderson, J.G. & Hoffman, P.D. 165
Gunderson, J.G. and Links, P. 42
Gunderson, J.G. et al. 74, 128, 131, 171

Hahn, T.N. 176
haloperidol, duration of use 141
happiness 182–3
harshness on self and others 17
Harvey, P. & Penzo, J.A. 164
Henderson, C. et al. 198
Henry, W.P. et al. 45
hierarchy of therapeutic areas 71–2
hippocampus 23
Hoffman, P.D. and Fruzzetti, A.E. 147, 168
Hoffman, P.D. et al. 169, 170
Hooley, J.M. and Hoffman, P.D. 148, 150
hopefulness 155
  clinicians 45
Horvath, A.O. and Bedi, R.P. 39, 47
Horvath, A.O. and Greenberg, L. 202
hospital admission *see* inpatient treatment
Huber, C. 185, 186
humility 161
humor 161
hurdles, chain analysis 197
hyperarousal, reduction strategies 192–3
hypersensitivity 104
hypervigilance 62

iatrogenesis 125–8
I-BAFT 171
idealization 9
identifying emotions 54, 95, 100–1
identity disturbance 9–10
identity group, DSM-IV-TR diagnostic
  criteria 14
identity issues 60
impact awareness 160
impulse control 101–3
impulsivity 60–1, 71
  DSM-IV-TR diagnostic criterion 10
impulsivity charts *102*
impulsivity group, DSM-IV-TR diagnostic
  criteria 14
information
  BPD handout for family and friends
    172–3
  on multisession family interventions 168
  provision to family and friends 147
  provision to patients 57–8
  reading list for friends and family 164–5
  useful websites 165–6
initial therapeutic stance 44–6

commonalities across generalist
treatments *37*
injustice, sensitivity to 17
inpatient treatment 124–5
impact on outcomes 125–8
indications for 128–34
purpose of admission 134–5
Integrative Borderline Adolescent Family
Therapy (I-BAFT) 171
International Classification of Diseases (ICD) 6
interpersonal effectiveness skills 200–1
interpersonal interactions 61–2, 71
DSM-IV-TR diagnostic criterion 9
group discussions 104–5
link to mood and emotions 99–100
interpersonal sensitivity 62
impact on therapeutic alliance 74–5
intervention types *81*
interviewing 81–2

JACOB acronym 188–92
joint crisis plans 198
consumer comment 198–9
Joyce, P.R. et al. 154
jumping to conclusions 190
Jurist, E.J. 177
justice, sense of 17

Karas, E. 39
Keller, M.B. et al. 128
Knaup, C. et al. 201
knowing versus non-knowing 85
koans 186
Kolla, N.J. et al. 52
Korzekwa, M.I. et al. 22
Krawitz, R. 45
Krawitz, R. & Jackson, W. 165
Kreger, R. 164
Kvarstein, E. & Karterud, S. 133

Lambert, M.J. and Barley, D.E. 46
lamotrigine 136
Laporte, L. and Guttman, H. 25
leadership 119
Lees, J. et al. 125
legal aspects, suicidal behavior 69–71
LeGris, J. 40
Leslie, A.M. 160
Linehan, M.M. 14, 18–19, 51–2, 113, 156–7,
170, 185, 193, 194
Lingiardi, V. et al. 74
links, chain analysis 196
Links, P. 40
listening 159
lithium 136
Lynch, T.R. et al. 83

maintenance medication 139–40

marking a task 121
Mason, B. 160
MBT-A 171
McCutcheon, L. 40
McFarlane, W.R. et al 146, 147
McLean Hospital program 171
McLean Study of Adult Development
(MSAD) 155
McMain, S. et al. 40
mechanisms of change 55
medication *see* prescribing
medication review 77, 133
Mental Health Act 70
mentalization-based therapy
accepting thoughts and valued action
187–8
chain analysis 194
comparison with SCM 39–40
decreasing hyperarousal 192–3
feedback 202
MBT-A 171
treatment outcome studies 32
mentalized affectivity 177
mentalizing 176–8
consumer comment 178–9
family/friend interventions 160–1
in team meetings 121
mentalizing teams 112, 115–16
mentalizing vulnerability 15
Miller, J. et al. 132–3
Miller, S.D. et al. 201
mindfulness 53, 176–8
consumer comment 178–9
misunderstandings 86
group discussions 104–5
monitoring of treatment 50–1
mood-dependent behaviour 11, 184
mood regulation 98–101, 136
morale, team support 118–19, 119–20
Moran, P. et al. 198
motivation for treatment 73–4
Multifamily DBT skills training 170
multisession interventions 143–4, 166–7
reading list 168
Munder, T. et al. 202

naltrexone 136
narcissistic personality disorder 132–3
National Education Alliance for BPD 165–6
nature and nurture interplay 25
Neacsiu, A.D. et al 55
Neff, K.D. 186
Neff, K.D. & Vonk, R. 192
Ng, F. et al. 201
NICE (National Institute for Health and
Clinical Excellence) guidelines
for family/friend interventions 145
for prescribing 135, 138, 142

Nistico, H. 40
nonattendance 73
  follow-up 152
  suicide risk 129
nonspecific interventions
  advocacy 89–90
  clinician attitude 82–6
  empathy 86–7
  interviewing 81–2
  positive regard 88–9
  validation 87–8
Norcross, J.C. 202
normalizing 159
Novick, J. 40

obesity, drug-related 141
obsessive–compulsive disorder 19
omega-3 fatty acids 136
opaqueness of mental states 160
openness of the clinician 83–4
open questions 81
opposite action strategies 96
organization willingness 45–6, 47
outcome feedback 201–2
Outcome Rating Scale 201, 202
outcome research, family/friend
    interventions 169–71
outlook 29–31, 155
overdose *see* self-harm
overgeneralizing 191

pain, "positive grieving" 151–2
panic disorder 19, 98
paranoid ideation 22, 104, 131–2
  antipsychotics 136
  DSM-IV-TR diagnostic criterion 12
paranoid personality disorder 23
parasuicide *see* self-harm
parenting
  DBT skills intervention 171
  management of emotional intensity 24
Paris, J. 42, 133
Parker, G. et al. 202
partners
  involvement in SCM 78–9
  role in crisis management 66
  teaching validation skills
    outcome research 171
  see also family/friend interventions
patient–clinician relationship *see* alliance
    ruptures; therapeutic alliance
patient expectations, relationship to
    treatment outcome 44
patient responsibilities 72–3
Penney, D. 170
Penney, D. & Woodward, P. 164–5
personality disorders
  characteristics 58–9

  emotion dysregulation 61
  impulsivity 60–1
  interpersonal interactions 61–2
  interpersonal sensitivity 62
  classification modifications 2, 6
  overlap 22–3
personality function, exploratory questions
    62–3
personalization 190
perspective-taking 160
pharmacological treatment outcome studies
    33
pharmacotherapy *see* prescribing
playfulness 161
"poorness of fit" concept 154, 155
Porr, V. 23, 153, 165, 168
"positive grieving" 151–2
positive regard 88–9
positive reinforcement, family/friend
    interventions 162
post-traumatic stress disorder 19, 21–2
Powers, M.B. et al. 179
practical problems, problem-solving
    approach 90–2
practical validation 159
pre-frontal cortex 153
prescribing 125, 135–7
  clinician cautions 137
  for comorbid conditions 141
  in crises 138–9
  discontinuation of medication 141
  discussion with the patient 140
  dosage 140
  duration of treatment 140–1
  guidelines 135, 142
  maintenance medication 139–40
  medication review 77, 133
prevalence of BPD 3, 26
primary emotions 93, 94–5, 184
private individual treatment 43
problem and solution analysis *see* chain
    analysis
problem behavior, chain analysis 195
problems, categorization of 92
problem-solving 199
problem-solving groups 90
  emotions, discussion of 92–8
  impulse control 101–3
  mood regulation 98–101
  practical problems 90–2
  on sensitivity and interpersonal problems
    104–5
  symptom reduction 92
prognosis 29–30, 155
  consumer comment 30–1
prompting events, chain analysis 195–6
psychodynamically based evidence-based
    treatments 32

psychoeducation 199
psychological mindedness 176
psychosocial treatment outcome studies 31–3
psychotherapy 31–3
   inpatient treatment, outcome study 127
   see also cognitive behavioral therapy;
      dialectical behavior therapy;
      structured clinical management
psychotic phenomena, interface with BPD
   21–2
psychotropic medication 135–7
   see also prescribing
public service team-based treatments 43
punishment 162

quality assurance 50–1
quality of treatment 36
questioning culture 120

Raes, F. 202
Rajalin, M. et al. 169
Rathus J.H. & Miller, A.L. 170
reasonable treatment 39
recovery 29–30
   consumer comment 30–1
reflecting upon emotions 96
reflective contemplation 160
regularity of scheduled sessions 50
reinforcement 82, 162
relapse rates 30
relationship difficulties 8, 60, 61–2, 104, 146
relationship management psychodynamic
   psychotherapy 32
relationship-mindfulness 178
relaxation techniques 97, 98
repetition of work 118
residential treatment *see* inpatient treatment
respect 117
responsibilities 161
risk assessment 68
   acute and chronic risk 68–9
   legal aspects 69–71
risky behavior 130
Roemer, E. & Orsillo, S.M. 176
Rossouw, T. 171

sadness 99–100, 182
safe uncertainty 160
scales analogy, treatment benefits 74
schema-focused therapy, treatment outcome
   study 32
schizophrenia, "expressed emotion" 148
screening questions 7–8
secondary emotions 93, 94–5, 184
selective serotonin reuptake inhibitors
   (SSRIs) 33, 135–6, 137
self-acceptance 184–6
   consumer comment 187

self-affect-state propositions 87
self-calming 193
self-care 162–3
self-compassion 52, 186
Self-Compassion Scale 202
self-criticism 94–5
self-esteem 185–6
self-harm 27
   approach in individual and group
      discussion 111
   causes 108–9
   consumer comments 28, 29
   correlation with suicide 29
   damage limitation 110
   definition 27, 106–7
   as a discriminating feature 13
   DSM-IV-TR diagnostic criterion 10–11
   emotional balancing properties 70
   interaction with treatment model 126, 127
   prevalence of BPD 4
   reduction strategies 109–10
   understanding of 27–9
   who does it? 108
   see also crisis planning; risk assessment
self-image, instability 9–10
self-loathing 185, 192
self-observation
   clients 53–4
   clinicians 52–3
self-reflection 103
self-reflective loop *177*
sensitivity 14–15, 24
   explanation to family members 153–4
   group discussions 104–5
sensitivity group, DSM-IV-TR diagnostic
   criteria 14
sensitivity reactions 131–2
separation anxiety 99
serotonin 23, 153
service organization 56–7
Session Rating Scale 202
severity, as a prognostic indicator 32
sexual abuse 4, 24–5, 26, 154
   involvement of family members/friends 149
Shearin, E.N. and Linehan, M.M. 45
Shimokawa, K. et al. 201
short intervention 150–66
signals, emotions as 100
Silk, K. 169
Skodol, A.E. 98–9
social phobia 19
social problems 72
   suicide risk 129
sociocultural factors in BPD 25
Soloff, P. et al. 141
specialist treatments
   indications for 54
   outcomes 31–2, 54–5

START criteria 121
step-down program, outcome study 126
stepping back 177
STEPPS (Systems Training for Emotional
    Predictability and Problem-solving)
    program 32, 169
Stone, M.H. 19, 127, 128
strategic processes 56
stress responses 182
structured clinical management (SCM) v,
    39–40, 57
    clinician and patient responsibilities 72–3
    comprehensive formulation 77–8
    core treatment strategies 80–1
        advocacy 89–90
        clinician attitude 82–6
        empathy 86–7
        impulse control 101–3
        interviewing 81–2
        mood regulation 98–101
        positive regard 88–9
        problem-solving groups 90–2
        self-harm 105–11
        sensitivity and interpersonal problems
            104–5
        tolerance of emotions 92–8
        validation 87–8
    crisis planning 65–8
    diagnosis communication 63–4
    explanation of treatment approach 78
    family/friend interventions 143–8
        multisession interventions 166–8
        short intervention 150–66
    hierarchy of therapeutic areas 71–2
    inpatient treatment 124–35
    involvement of friends and family 78–9
    medication stabilization 77
    motivation 73–4
    prescribing 135–42
    risk assessment 68–71
    substance abuse 76
    team meetings 120–1
    teamwork 112–23
    therapeutic alliance 74–5
structure of treatment 49, 57–8
substance abuse 76, 132
    and BDP diagnosis 4
    co-occurrence with BPD 20, 61, 98
suicidal behavior 20–1
    DSM-IV-TR diagnostic criterion 10–11
    legal aspects 69–71
    management of 53
    see also self-harm
suicide risk
    acute risk 124
    assessment of 68–9, 129–30
    impact of other personality disorders
        132–3

relationship to hopelessness 45
relationship to self-harm 29, 106–7, 109
suicides, effect on clinicians 119
supervision of clinicians 51–2, 122–3
    dealing with likes and dislikes 89
support groups 150–1
supportive psychotherapy (SP) 41
sympathy, distinction from empathy 87
symptom reduction, problem-solving
    approach 92

target areas 78
team meetings 120–1
teamwork 51–2, 112
    mentalizing 115–16
    mutual support 118–19
    rationale 113–15
    supervision 122–3
    sustaining enthusiasm 119–20
    united mind 116–18
telephone contact 73
therapeutic alliance 46–8, 48, 74–5
    commonalities across generalist
        treatments 37
    Division 29 Task Force on Empirically
        Supported Therapy Relationships
        46–7
    empathy and validation 49
    feedback 202
    parallels with supervision relationships,
        122–3
    see also alliance ruptures
therapeutic areas, hierarchy of 71–2
thoughts
    acceptance of 187
    JACOB acronym 188–92
time-frames 50
topiramate 136
Torgersen, S. et al. 24, 153
transference-focused therapy
    comparison with SP and DBT 41
    treatment outcome studies 32
trauma, "positive grieving" 151–2
treatment aspects
    initial therapeutic stance 44–6
    therapy relationship 46–9
    treatment model features 37, 49–53
treatment benefits, scales analogy 74
treatment details, sources 43
treatment modules 92
treatment outcomes, historical background 3
treatment outcome studies
    pharmacological treatments 33
    psychosocial treatments 31–3
treatment recommendations 41–3
treatment strategies 175–6
    accepting thoughts and valued action
        187–8

chain analysis 193–8
changing thoughts 188–92
decreasing hyperarousal 192–3
discussion with the patient 78
mentalizing and mindfulness 176–9
outcome feedback 201–2
self-acceptance 184–7
skills
   DBT distress tolerance skills 200
   DBT interpersonal effectiveness skills
     200–1
structure
   joint crisis plans 198–9
   problem-solving 199
   psychoeducation 199
summary 174–5
valued action irrespective of emotions
   179–80
   acceptance of emotions 181–2
   identification of emotions 182–4
Trull, T.J. et al. 76
trusting attitude 161
Tryon, G.S. and Winograd, G. 48
"turning the mind" 185
turn-taking 161
twin studies 24, 153
two-session interventions 143, 150–66
Tyrer, P. & Bateman, A. 128, 137

validation of clients 49, 87–8
   DBT structuring 159
   family/friend interventions 155–7
   outcome research 171
   personal description 158
validation of clinicians 52
valued action 179–80, 184, 187–8
   consumer comment 180
van Gelder, K. *20*
van Wel, B. et al. 169
Vermote, R. et al. 127
violence, risk to partners 146
vulnerability factors, chain analysis 195

warmth, conveyance of 88–9
warning signs for crises 65–6
Weinberg, I. et al. 42–3, 47
welcoming of clients 45, 47–8
well-structured treatment 49
Wenzel, A. et al. 44, 51, 202
Widom, C.S. et al. 25, 154
Working Alliance Inventory 202
Wright, J.H. et al. 45, 194
Wupperman, P. et al. 53

Zanarini, M.C. 39, 42
Zanarini, M.C. et al. 25, 29–30, 127–8, 139, 141
Zen, koans 186